# You Only Live Thrice

## Perspective is a Superpower

Karl Perry

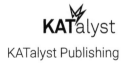

KATalyst

KATalyst Publishing

Published in 2021 by KATalyst Publishing

ISBN Paperback: 978-1-7398563-0-4
ISBN Ebook: 978-1-7398563-1-1

A CIP catalogue copy of this book can be found in the British Library.

Front cover design by Karl Perry. Artwork by Jansen Yee

**Disclaimer**

This book is a memoir - a work of non-fiction based on the experiences and recollections of the author.

Except in such minor respects not affecting the substantial accuracy of the work, the contents of this book are true. Names of medical individuals have been changed. Names of the institutions have been removed.

Any opinions of people, processes, systems or institutions mentioned in this book are based on the author's experience during the period specified. It is recognised that others may have different opinions or experiences with those people, processes, systems or institutions.

The author's experience is that of a patient and is not medically trained. Medical references such as conditions, symptoms, procedures, and pharmaceutical solutions should not be used as guidance. This book is not intended as a substitute for the medical advice of physicians. The reader should consult a physician in matters relating to his/her health and particularly with respect to any symptoms similar to those referenced in this book.

On the other hand, if you really need to be told that, you deserve what you get!

KATalyst Publishing, 2021

To Karina, George and Ben: Love you more.
For Mum & Dad: You showed me the true meaning of
persistence, resilience and strength.

*Fate whispers to the warrior,*
*'You cannot withstand the storm.'*

*The warrior whispers back,*
*'I am the storm.'*
**Unknown**

# CONTENTS

# CONTENTS

CONTENTS

# Begintroduction

*"Change isn't a four-letter word...*
*but often your reaction to it is."*
**Jeffrey Gitomer**

I just want to make one thing very clear. When I first started to write in December 2020, I had absolutely no intention of writing a book. It had never crossed my mind to write a book and if it had, I wouldn't have known how to write a book. So, having never written a book before, I had no idea about the process or if there was some secret technique authors use. Do they plan everything out and know exactly where they're going before they start or just write what they're thinking at the time and put it all in some sort of order afterwards? But all of that was irrelevant - because I wasn't planning on writing a book.

The undeniable truth though, is you appear to be holding something bearing a remarkable likeness to a book, which unquestionably has my name on the front. So how did we get from one state of affairs to the other? A good question and one I've frequently asked myself. The honest answer is, I'm not entirely sure except to say, this book is simply the by-product of a process I discovered I was working through. It was never the goal. There never really was a goal. I just had to get a lot of stuff out of my head and the easiest way to do it was to write it down.

You deserve an explanation.

Prior to 2019, my life had felt relatively in order. As much as most people's, I guess. Not without challenges but pretty good. I'd just turned 50 years old, had been married to my lovely wife, Karina, for 21 years and had two fantastic teenage lads who'd brought no trouble to our door. I owned and ran my own event management agency. There were no Porsches on the drive, but no wolf at the door either. I was healthy, active, had plenty of great mates and was generally enjoying life. If only Manchester United could learn to be consistent over *both* halves of a game.

During the spring of 2019, all four wheels fell off my life when I had a sudden cardiac arrest at home. I'm writing this, so you'll know I survived. I've never been so grateful for anything in my life. I'm not glossing over it. I'll take you through the whole, warts n all, detailed story. Some might say *too* detailed, but I'd struggle to feel my account was authentic if you don't feel the need to cringe at certain points. I did at the time and still do now.

I eventually returned to work but I was glad to see the back of 2019. 2020 then started badly with my Mum dying and continued to unravel. By any measure, 2020 was an arsehole of a year. A confusing, disastrous, life-changingly shit, arsehole of a year. Covid-19 swept across the globe, upending lives, families, and society in general, regardless of country.

I've never been a great sleeper, but that year had been vintage in the insomnia stakes, although I generally had no trouble getting off to sleep. It was staying asleep which had always been the problem.

I used to call them the '4 am demons', waking me and hijacking my mind for 2-3 hours. Mostly they were never particularly demonic, although I felt like hell by the time I had to get out of bed and start the day. But towards the end of 2020, as was probably the case for many, the 4 am demons were putting in longer days, arriving earlier and partying later. A lot of it was just space junk floating around; things I had to do; things to continue doing; parts of conversations that may have happened or may yet happen. So mostly, space junk.

I say *mostly* because, towards the end of the year, a thread had begun to appear. Words and phrases were gradually converging, and thoughts were beginning to form like embryonic clumps of cells.

I began to think something was happening to me. Which was a bit weird, because by then, I'd thought something had *already* happened to me. Something, or more accurately, *things* – those things I've just mentioned had happened, but they quite firmly resided in the past tense. They were things I'd gotten over, accepted with my usual level of resilience (which even if I say so myself, is quite considerable), and I'd moved on from.

But by the end of the year, these embryonic bits of something had broken through into the daylight hours and I was becoming unsettled by them. I wasn't sure where they were taking me or why I was giving them oxygen, but I had to find out what was going on.

Of course, there were some winners in the pandemic. There had to be. But for many, 2020 will go down as one of the direst years in recent human history. Personally, one of the low lights was having to close the event management business I'd been building and investing in over the previous 15 years. Pretty desperate stuff. But that's not the worst thing that had happened to me over the 12 months prior to the onset of the pandemic. Dying (albeit temporarily) at home due to my cardiac arrest and being resuscitated by my wife would definitely rank higher. Losing my Mum at the start of 2020 was devastating too and would arguably also pitch in above the loss of my business.

I used this '*not the worst thing*' phrase quite a bit as 2020 unfolded. It helped provide some perspective on the shitstorm going on all around me, all year long. And it's worth clarifying: I *closed* the business. It hadn't gone bust. More on this later but it had been a controlled exit and therefore arguably far less traumatic than the scenarios forced upon thousands of other businesses during 2020.

So, what was the issue?

I'd thought I'd dealt with the events of the previous 18 months, but by December 2020, those embryonic murmurings suggested that may not have been the case. Getting this stuff out and on to paper, or through a keyboard at least, was my attempt to review the events of those previous 18 months. To try and make sense of them; of the thoughts and feelings generated by them, and to try and get a grip on what the hell was going on in my mind.

Much to my total surprise, the process has been hugely cathartic. Eventually, by capturing an account of this phase of my life, I began to realise what my subconscious had been trying to get through to me: that the Universe had gifted me something priceless. In its simplest terms, I'd been given the wondrous and wonderful prize of the unknown. Ahead of me lay the potential and the opportunity for new beginnings; a blank canvas ready for a fresh adventure; a chance to press the reset button. Call it what you will.

By the close of 2020, I hadn't consciously appreciated that this was the case. But something in my subconscious, reptilian brain was telling me that in failing to recognise it, I was in danger of wasting the opportunity of a new direction. If surviving the cardiac arrest was the start of a second life, then a totally blank canvas was surely a third incarnation of life. I just had to try and work out what that would look like, which in honesty, is still a work in progress. This shouldn't be a surprise to me. Part of the joy of stacking up the years is realising that we're all work in progress. There's no finish line.

Mine isn't an isolated journey. Many people will have experienced the things I have. Certainly, the death of a parent is almost hard-wired into life. Although admittedly, being sandwiched between your own death and the death of your company is a stretch from the norm.

But having gone through the process, I've inadvertently ended up with this book. I don't know if it's a good book. It's certainly very honest. Brutal in parts and I'm told, funny in others. It's a memoir for sure, although I think the human condition is universal and parallels can be drawn in dealing with life's challenges, regardless of what they are for each of us individually.

In revisiting those 18 months I took away three key lessons. Perspective is a superpower and goes a long way in coping with life's more challenging phases. I suggest deploying it daily, hourly, whenever needed. Be your own catalyst. Secondly, celebrate the small wins. Too many look for the big win. The reality is, the biggest win is the accumulation of all the little wins.

I think most of all though, getting through tough times is about having hope. It can feel irrational at times when presented with contrary facts, truth, and reality. But the fact, the truth and the reality is, that life will take its course and bad times *will* inevitably happen. But how you *feel* during those bad times, shall eventually pass.

Actually, I've just thought of a fourth key lesson: no matter what the reason for your hospital stay, accept that your genitals won't come through it unscathed.

So, in keeping with the theme of hope, I hope after reading this far, you feel inclined to continue and won't be disappointed to discover 'You Only Live Thrice' isn't a James Bond sequel. (Aren't they all?) It's about many things; a patient's account of surviving cardiac arrest, definitely; but much wider than that, it's about recognising signposts when the Universe puts them in front of you and understanding the potential for those signposts. And you don't have to experience any kind of trauma to do that. You can begin the lookout for signposts and their potential, right this second. Who knows what opportunities may unfold, if we looked at things a little differently, made decisions we wouldn't usually make or occasionally moved closer to the edge of our comfort zones? We all have more input in the direction of our lives than we ever give ourselves credit for.

Just before I continue, it's probably worth saying there will be a few medical terms and procedures referenced throughout these rambles and I can't assume everyone will understand them. I sometimes still struggle, myself. As such, I'll always attempt to provide a brief layman's explanation. By way of a caveat though, my *York Notes* summations should not be compared with anything to be found in *Gray's Anatomy* and should under no circumstances be used as a means of self-diagnosis.

That's what Google is for.

You'll remember your teachers at school telling you a story should have a beginning, a middle and an end? In some respects, the end is yet to be written, but then that's the point of the tale. So that also makes it kind of hard to define a middle. However, there is probably a fairly identifiable start to the story, which takes us back to March 1st 2019, so it makes sense for the opening scene to be set there.

Buckle up.

# 2

## Bells & Whistles

*"Fall down seven times, get up eight."*

**Japanese Proverb**

It's probably abnormal to be excited about going into hospital for a procedure requiring an overnight stay. It wasn't the *8yr-old-kid-coming-down-on-Christmas-morning-to-discover-a-bike* kind of excitement, but there was definitely a sense of nervous anticipation. I'd like to say it was because I knew the procedure would secure me a safer future, but if I was being honest, it was more that it was happening at one of South Manchester's most respected private hospitals. I'm just a bang average bloke from Costa del Cleethorpes and had never had a procedure in a private hospital before. The prospect of the additional *bells & whistles* I'd heard about, had put a spring in my step. (I know. I'm so deep.) That – and the fact my company medical insurance was covering the cost of said bells & whistles.

Remarkably, I was totally lacking in any kind of fear or trepidation usually associated with surgery. Possibly because the procedure was elective, (and therefore not life or death). Or maybe it was because my Cardiologist, let's call him Dr A, was so convincingly reassuring; both in terms of the success rate of the procedure (c.80%) and the unlikelihood of collateral damage, such as death or stroke. Which was nice.

I trusted him implicitly from a clinical point of view. But Dr A also had more than a passing resemblance to Sting, the tantric Rock-God and possessed the most calming voice I've ever heard come out of a human being. His bedside manner was woven from pure silk. If he'd told me, as a precaution, prior to the procedure, he'd have to remove my bollocks, I would've seen the upside. As Sade would have said, he was a Smooth Operator.

All these factors fed into my complete lack of anxiety as I strolled past the uniformed doorman, welcoming patients into the building as though we'd be washing down lobster with a 1953 Dom Perignon within 20 minutes. With hindsight, I wonder if I was in some form of denial about the seriousness of the game in which I'd found myself a player. Not one that I, or anyone, would ever choose to take part in, but like Jumanji, once started, there's no packing up and walking away. Mine was to be a lifelong game that had started at the end of 2016 when I'd been diagnosed with a heart condition called Atrial Fibrillation – AF for short.

For those unfamiliar with AF, in its simplest terms, it's a condition that causes an irregular and often fast heartbeat. Essentially, it's caused by flaws in the electrical circuitry of the heart and can cause a patient to feel breathless on exertion. Left untreated, AF can lead to blood clots, stroke, heart failure and other heart-related complications, which in turn, unsurprisingly, can lead to death.

I'll leave it there with the science but whereas a healthy heart should sing to the tune of:
Dum-dum...dum-dum...dum-dum... (a sinus rhythm)
Mine had developed a more inconsistent and less melodic rhythm:
Dum...dum-dum-dum...........dum-dum... dum-dum-dum-dum-dum.... (more like morse code)

The procedure I was not in the least bit afraid of having, was a *catheter ablation*. The aim of which was to restore my heart to a normal sinus rhythm and heart rate. Anything in the 60-80 bpm range would be good, rather than the 100+ I usually experienced, even sitting down.

'What on earth is a catheter ablation?' I hear you murmur. Well, I think I'm right in saying it involves passing thin, flexible tubes, called catheters, through the blood vessels to the heart. The catheters identify the heart's electrical activity and so can pinpoint where it's going wrong. Alarmingly, the area affected is then destroyed using heat or by freezing which causes scarring, which doesn't allow the erroneous electricity to pass through. The idea is that the heart's electrical activity reverts to the correct circuitry. Apologies for the simplicity to anyone who really does know what they're talking about.

It's often the way with heart conditions that they tend *not* to occur in isolation. They're usually caused by, or cause other coronary related issues and sure enough, as we'd gone through the diagnostics, another was discovered in the form of moderate regurgitation of my Mitral Valve. Discovering one of my heart valves was being sick, · caused me some alarm.

Naturally, Dr A bathed me in reassurance. Apparently, it was nowhere near the stage where they would consider operating. His thinking was that if we could get the AF under control, it would greatly help with the performance of the valve. Incidentally, valve regurgitation just means the valve is allowing backflow of blood into the chamber that should have emptied. I'm not sure why I used the word *just*. If you want to generate blood clots in the heart, this is one of the most effective ways to do it.

Although the Police frontman had raised the option of the catheter ablation, he couldn't categorically say he thought the procedure was necessary. An unusual stance for a Doctor and as a patient,

I've never really been a fan of treatment bordering on the unnecessary. His dilemma was that I was asymptomatic and fully active. Whilst he couldn't guarantee an ablation would resolve the AF, if it did, then it could potentially reduce the risk of blood clots and stroke in later life. Equally, it could cause one on the operating table, but that only happened in about one in a thousand cases. Naturally, I enquired what number he was at since the last stroke. Apparently, it didn't work like that.

Deciding on elective procedures isn't usually an easy thing. By their nature, they're not critical and they come with risks; but then there is the potential for the upside. It wasn't lost on me that my Dad had a stroke aged 61 and died at 63 due to left ventricular failure. I was otherwise fit and healthy: it would either work or it wouldn't. The risks were minimal and the most reassuring man on the planet was at the wheel, or the scalpel or whatever it was they use.

And so, it was decided: let's try and make the future safer for ourselves and if it doesn't work, it doesn't work. I'd be no worse off. Where do I sign?

Back to March 1st 2019. Once I'd checked in (their phrase, not mine), I was directed to my private room with ensuite bathroom, large wall-mounted TV, a hot drinks tray, a proper wardrobe and an overnight bag rack. I'd stayed in hotel rooms with fewer facilities. I was given the usual gown but also a set of snazzy elasticated, baggy disposable pants. Not what you'd call *pulling pants* but very functional in terms of dignity protection. The bells were a-ringing. Within no time I was wheeled away in a chair, towards the theatre.

Dr A and an Anaesthetist were casually leaning against something I hoped wasn't too important, talking football. I found their relaxed demeanour comforting to the point where I wanted to join in but wasn't sure I could pull off blokey banter given they would shortly be up close and personal with my genitals, as the incision was to be in the femoral artery in my groin.

Within seconds I'm onto the table and under a heated blanket with the Anaesthetist asking me to count slowly backwards from ten. I held a picture of Karina and the kids in my mind during the countdown but became concerned when I'd got to four. I didn't want to tell him his job which was fortunate, as three never arrived.

Within what felt like a blink, I was coming around, back in my own room and breathing through an oxygen mask. Karina was beside me and in no time at all, I was feeling good. Really good. The mask was removed. I sat up and was asked if I wanted a cup of tea and anything to eat. I was very hungry given I'd had to skip breakfast and was passed a lunch menu a gastropub would have been proud of. In the distance, there may have been the faint euphony of bells & whistles.

Naturally, I was keen to know how the procedure had gone, so whilst waiting for my starter, I'd asked my nurse. Apparently, Dr A would be able to explain. This wasn't the immediate reassurance I was hoping for but was told he'd be along in about 20 minutes. My faith in him was absolute and besides, my seafood risotto starter had just arrived so that took my mind off the wait.

By the time the Police frontman (seeing as he was a *Sting-a-like*, let's call him Gordon) arrived, I was just finishing my Chicken Arrabbiata, so it had been a little longer than the suggested 20 minutes, but I certainly wasn't counting. The sauce was gorgeous and somewhere, there was a New York cheesecake with my name on it.

'Hello, Karl. How are you feeling?'

'Hi, Gordon.' I wasn't being disrespectful dropping his professional title. I think when someone has been up that close to your groin, then being on first name terms is the very least you can expect. In fact, if anything, as a Surgeon, his title should really be *Mister*, to distinguish himself from *Doctor*. I've always thought it a typically British quirk of snobbery, that in days of yore, whilst you still had to train to earn the title of Doctor, anyone could have a go at surgery, hence Surgeons were only allowed the title of Mister. (And probably never a Mrs or Ms.) But I digress.

'So how did it go?' I asked as I dabbed my mouth with the linen napkin.

'Very well. The procedure was a technical success.'

Was a *technical success* an *actual success* or the opposite of success but heavily spun, my face clearly must have asked. Gordon smiled, so I knew it was going to be okay.

'A sinus rhythm was achieved but then reverted back to AF,' he said. 'I did further work and we got another sinus rhythm but you reverted back again. I don't want to do any more work at this point as it's not uncommon to jump in and out different rhythms following ablation. You've got to remember, your heart has never been touched before, so it's a bit bruised right now. It can sometimes take up to six weeks before a sinus rhythm is properly settled.'

Now – this potential outcome of a delayed result wasn't made especially clear to me in our earlier meetings, so I can't lie, I felt somewhat disappointed. I'd expected to be told it had either worked or it hadn't. Gordon continued to stress he was confident a favourable outcome was still very likely. I just had to be patient and rest for the next few days. The most important thing at that point was to let the incision in my groin seal. I was to move as little as possible and use bottles for the toilet, until the morning. Whilst I really wanted to believe him about the ultimate outcome, the cheesecake just didn't taste quite as good as I'd hoped.

By that point, I hadn't even checked under my gown, so once Gordon had left, I carried out a full inspection. Unsurprisingly, the snazzy pants had been removed. A thick, padded dressing was heavily taped to the right of my nutbag, pushing everything to port. Just the tiniest dot of dark red was visible in the middle of the square white gauze. And speaking of nutbags, this one no longer looked like mine.

Larger, definitely. Smoother and shinier, undeniably. And purply-black in colour, suggesting some kind of violent assault had taken place. Just looking at them caused an involuntary grimace, quickly followed by the realisation that I couldn't feel any pain. The anaesthetic was still doing its job so I filed those oversized shiny bad-boys under *not to worry for now – review later*. I could only surmise that, in order to cut into my femoral artery to insert the catheter, my bollocks had to be clamped into something akin to a school metal-work vice.

The *not getting out of bed and hardly moving* instruction was not difficult to follow. The TV was on and there seemed to be a nurse asking if I wanted a cup of tea every 45 mins. Biscuits and snacks were brought, followed by the menu for the evening meal. I maxed it out. Anything that came my way – I was in. I went for the whole shooting match: foil-wrapped biscuits, more tea, crisps, more tea, shortbread, more tea, more tea, more tea... ahhh the sweet sound of those bells & whistles. Eventually, inevitably, I needed a wee. Badly.

Now, there is an art to successfully carrying out the male-bed-bottle procedure. It can take a few attempts before you learn to avoid a Code Yellow scenario. Certainly, the anticipated challenge of the first attempt tends to encourage deferment. In my case, I was all but in Apollo 13 territory.

Everything about weeing in bed feels wrong. (Or it should do.) Am I in? Is the angle right? Gravity is against you. And then relaxing enough to let go. Although being in Apollo 13 territory helps. Once in flow, concern switches to, staying inside the bottle; is it tilting too much? Am I going to pour it over myself? (To be avoided at all costs given the implications for sheet changes when told not to move.)

All those cups of tea meant I could've put out an Ozzie bushfire. Then came the fear. There's a change in tone as the liquid approached the neck of the bottle. Shit – it was getting full, and I needed to cut off. I was looking under the sheets trying to balance the equation between how much space was left and how much more I felt I was going to expel. Fortunately, shutdown occurs with some breathing space, although not much.

But, and this is crucial when that part of a man's body is in the neck of the bottle, there is very little shake room. No man wants an unwelcome follow-up. If standing up, this would go down the trouser leg. (Otherwise known as a *Wembley* – the longest dribble on the pitch.)

With the control and dexterity of a bomb-disposal expert, I attempted the manoeuvre, whilst trying not to shake the bottle too much and induce spillage or disturb my dressing. I failed on the spillage front and then Wembley'd anyway. It wasn't a huge amount, so I traded off a small damp patch with not having to embarrass myself with the nurses. (It's only a Code Yellow if you tell them.) It seemed a reasonable trade-off, but mental notes were made regarding future performances. Apollo 13 territory was to be avoided at all costs and I decided to cut back on the tea for a few hours.

I was making the most of the facilities and was enjoying flicking through the TV channels. There was nothing on I wanted to watch, but by that time it was 9:30 pm and what I did want to do, was squeeze every last drop from the comfortable facilities provided. So, my supper of cheese and biscuits, washed down with two cups of tea, was accompanied by a re-run of *the 100 most embarrassing celebrity moments of 2018.*

After a very short time, the sheer excitement of the day was weighing on me and I knew I had to think about getting some sleep. Naturally, a wee before bedtime wouldn't go amiss but I was getting a bit concerned about the damp patch between my legs. Each time I'd used a bottle, there had been some sort of Wembley occurrence. I was keen to avoid compounding this situation, so decided to sit on the edge of the bed to use the carafe.

I shuffled myself round and was fully sitting up. I positioned the bottle and noticed that the little red dot on the dressing was a little bigger but thought that was to be expected. I'm not sure why exactly I thought that was to be expected, given my medical training only went as far as putting someone in the recovery position for a Scout badge. I pulled the bedsheet over the whole enterprise, as my room door was open, and I wasn't in a position to pull the curtain around. I didn't really want to be on view should a nurse suddenly walk in. I then relaxed and enjoyed the most satisfying release of the day.

I squeezed slightly to make sure everything was out. As I did, a noise became apparent. It was the sound of liquid pouring onto the floor. I simultaneously had a very warm, wet feeling between my legs and buttocks. I instantly knew that somehow, despite thinking it had all gone to plan, I'd pissed myself, big style. 'Shit,' I thought. 'Now they'll *have* to change the sheets.'

I pulled back the bedsheet used to protect my modesty and froze. In no way was I prepared for the sight that greeted me. In the cup created by the dip of me sitting on the edge of the bed, with my thighs being the edges, was a deep pool of very dark red liquid, over-flowing onto the floor and splashing loudly and widely. I was quite literally stunned. I had no pain but felt confusion and shock. It felt like ages but must have only been a few seconds before I reached for the call button on the table. In doing so, the pool between my legs tilted forward and poured even more of the dark red stuff onto the floor.

I screamed for a nurse a couple of times and one arrived after about 10 seconds. I have no recollection of what she shouted but within seconds there were three of them and within a minute I had four nurses and a Doctor around my bed.

The bed was inverted backwards as far as it would go, so my head was way lower than my feet, with the aim of keeping the blood still within my body, within my body. The tilted bed caused the blood on the bed to run down my back, neck and into my armpits. In what seemed to be one move, the Doctor ripped off the dressing and rammed his elbow into my groin sealing the incision. Despite his speed, there was just enough time for a single spurt of blood to arc into the air and land on my body. It was probably a relatively small amount, but it made a hell of a splash.

Urgent instructions were hastily exchanged. A bag of saline was connected to the cannula in my hand. A blood pressure cuff was attached. Nurses shuffled positions. I was repeatedly asked if I was OK and remarkably, I felt fine. It was a most surreal sight and although I felt no panic, there was clearly a very real danger, hence the response. Bleeding out, can, I suppose, be classed as something of a dangerous scenario. I was clearly in shock.

My head was between knee and thigh height and whilst I couldn't see much of what was going on, I could see the floor. It was alien to me, as a real-world sight. The blood from the original splash site was, by then, spread all around my bed in the form of Croc footprints and slip marks from the Doctor's shoes. I was on a set from a Tarantino film.

Activity eventually stabilised. One nurse retreated and another went in search of a mop and bucket to clean the floor. This left two nurses and Dr Elbow. It was only about 15 minutes since the whole thing had started but for me, it had been an age. The medical emergency had subsided. I'd remained completely stable and everything that could've been done, had been done. The conversation lightened a little as the remaining three, fixed to their posts, made comments about the *most embarrassing moments* programme still going on in the background. Suddenly, the nurse on my left turned to me and said, 'I'm really sorry to have to be doing this. I hope I'm not hurting you.'

I was still inverted and still in shock and so, not really engaged with the room. As such, I hadn't really clocked that this nurse had my already engorged genitals in her hand and was pulling them very firmly over to the left, allowing the Doctor enough space to get his elbow into my groin. As first dates go, this one was moving fast. At this rate, we'd be in Ikea picking Billy units for our apartment, by sunrise.

'No, not at all,' I replied, wishing desperately I could've come up with something so incredibly witty, she'd be struggling to breathe when recounting the story to friends and family.

Although, I did make a mental note to take T'pau's *China in Your Hands* off my playlist.

After 45 minutes, an even larger pressure dressing was taped over the wound and into my groin. I was cleaned up, the sheets changed and the multiple Wembleys a distant memory. I was exhausted by then and went to sleep quickly but not without first skimming through the rushes of the previous hour or so. Apparently, I'd been in real danger. But what I couldn't get out of my mind was, for 45 minutes, a nurse's only job had been to hold my bollocks. I'm sure had the same situation occurred in an NHS hospital, the same processes and procedures would have been followed. But probably not whilst watching *most embarrassing moments*.

In terms of the whole story, this particular incident plays absolutely no part, except to say that upon being discharged the following day, I was very much of the mind that my faith in Dr A was absolute and the necessity for any further intervention with my heart was over. The drama was done, and so, as Yazz would have said, the only way was up.

# 3

# Lemsips

*"If you fall, I'll always be there."*
**The Floor**

February to June was always the busiest time of year for Assured Events, my event management agency. Every 2-3 weeks there'd be a 2-4 day conference with an exhibition and various themed and awards dinners attached. Coupled with setup and breakdown days and the four bank holidays during that period, it always made for a demanding and stressful phase of the year. We all steeled ourselves for it, but it never got any easier, despite recruiting more staff, as we'd also win additional business each year.

The usual business issues would also arise; payment chasing; dealing with 3$^{rd}$ party incompetence; government red tape... all the bollocks which made you wonder why you even bothered in the first place.

The previous summer, unbeknownst to the wider team, I'd started a conversation with our Account Director, essentially my deputy in the company, about her possibly buying me out, known imaginatively as a Management Buy Out (MBO). She was interested but exploring the deal was taking a great deal of our attention and time, in addition to the running of the business and planning and delivering our clients' events.

I'd been thinking of some sort of exit for a while. Maybe it was age or maybe I was becoming tired of the cyclical nature of recruiting and developing people, only for some to realise just how demanding working in an event agency is. And of clients increasingly expecting more for less (or at least for no more). It was all beginning to wear a bit thin. I was hugely proud of what we'd created and we were well respected within the industry. But by then, it no longer made my heart sing. It no longer allowed me to feel like me at my best and I no longer had the same energy levels. Or if I had, I just couldn't channel them into the company the way I could in the past. I knew I had to get out.

Everyone looks at the company owner and thinks *hey, they've got it made – they can do what they want!* Well, there may be perks, but unlike every other employee, I had no contractual clause I could point to and say, *I'm out!* I felt trapped. I couldn't give the job my best because the job wasn't allowing me to be me. The slow pace of the MBO was also frustrating, but understandable given the workload we were under. This all weighed heavy on me. I tried not to show it but Karina knew me too well. She knew the toll it was taking on me, even if, outwardly, the rest of the world thought all was well in the House of Karl.

So, it was against this backdrop that, two weeks after the ablation and redecoration of my private hospital room, we were going away for a couple of days and a night to Kirkby Lonsdale in Yorkshire with some close friends. It was a birthday gift for my 50^th, the previous December and our friends were treating us to a meal and overnight stay in an old coaching inn.

I'd taken on board Gordon's comments that it may take up to six weeks for a sinus rhythm to be established. It hadn't at that point –

I was still in AF. Although there were still four of the six weeks left, I was disappointed there'd been no improvement. The truth was, I was feeling worse than before the ablation. I'd been warned my heart would be sore after the procedure but would settle down. We'd also discussed the 80% likelihood of success (so it was never guaranteed), but at no point did we ever have the discussion that I could end up feeling worse than before the ablation.

It's worth qualifying what I mean by worse. Prior to the AF, if I checked my pulse, it was irregular; no dum-dum... dum-dum... dum-dum... for me. However, I'd never got breathless going upstairs or on hill walks. I could cycle, exercise and go about my normal life with no impairment. I was classed as asymptomatic. By then though, activity was more of an effort. Breathing was more laboured. I could feel my heart having to work harder when engaging in even modestly raised activity levels.

During the visit to Kirkby Lonsdale, we went for a walk along the river just outside the village. It was a real slog and I feigned excuses to stop whether to take in a view or have a water break. We'd set ourselves a particular route and at one stage followed the river with a view to crossing a bridge we could see on the map. There was a slight incline to get there and the ground was a little heavy. I could feel my heart labouring. When we got to the footbridge it was closed for repair so we'd have to head back 25 minutes to the village, cross the road bridge there and go up the river on the other side to continue our route.

The thought of adding another 50 minutes onto what was a leisurely walk, caused me both anger and distress, neither of which I shared. I was angry because I didn't want to do it, as well as angry that I felt angry. I was distressed because I wasn't entirely sure I could even physically do it. By the time we'd got to the road bridge, I declared my hand, said I was tired and had had enough. I murmured something about it being the first exercise I'd done since the ablation and didn't want to push it. There was probably more surprise than was shown, but then everyone was also quite happy to head back to the Inn and settle by the fire. We'd only been walking for an hour.

What had happened to me? This wasn't the me I recognised. A few weeks prior I'd been happily cycling in the foothills of the Peak District; rushing around at events, helping with setups, carrying boxes; going for walks, There's something fundamentally unnerving when your body suddenly doesn't perform at the levels you expect. A bubble of fear begins to swell.

This too was beginning to weigh heavy on me.

By Saturday 13th April it was the magic six weeks since my ablation. I hadn't noticed any improvement in my condition. I was still in AF for sure. But activity-wise, I was still in a worse place than before the ablation. I hadn't healed at all.

Outwardly, I doubt anyone realised. But it'd got to the stage where I noticed I wasn't looking forward to taking the two flights of stairs to our office, and with good reason. I might linger a while once at the top, just to catch a few breaths. Walking down the High Street at lunch might entail looking in a few more shop windows than usual. I was no longer cycling or walking at weekends.

We had an event in Lancaster running from Sunday 14th to Wednesday 17th April but the project team of five had gone ahead on the 13th to set up. I was keen to avoid joining them that day for a number of reasons: the sheer effort and energy the setting up would require; event management was losing its lustre for me (whereas I'd previously loved the buzz of working away and setting up amazing client experiences), but also quite crucially, my eldest son George, was playing in a rugby final in Widnes on Sunday 14th.

The project team were more than capable of handling the setup and my plan was to drive up from Widnes to Lancaster following the game on the Sunday. I was so tired on the Saturday afternoon whilst I was packing. Karina said to me, 'Are you ok? You look grey.' I answered with absolute honesty when I replied, 'I feel grey.' I was washed-out and bereft of energy. In her most wifely of tones, she told me to have a power nap. I didn't argue.

I woke feeling so much more refreshed the following day. George won his final and I met the project team in Lancaster with everything already in place for that evening. Once the event was underway, there were times I had to get my hands dirty and help with moving kit, which required effort beyond the usual. It was a large event site too, so we were easily covering 25-30,000 steps some days. We were up at 6 am and going to bed at gone 1 am and as long as those days were, it wasn't always easy to drop off to sleep quickly. If I was getting four hours, that was a result.

Tuesday night was the final evening and the awards dinner. Typically, on the last night of an event, the team would have a couple of glasses of wine, recognising the job was nearly done and the demands were lifting. The team kept with tradition, but I'd started on the Lemsips earlier that afternoon so didn't bother with the wine or even feel like being there at all.

I was headachy, lethargic and when I took in a really big breath, I felt a coldness in my lungs. It wasn't an ache, and it wasn't there when breathing normally. It crossed my mind about a possible link to my AF, but I suspected some sort of mild bug. It certainly didn't stop me from working.

I continued the Lemsips the following morning and lunchtime, after which, the conference concluded. I arrived home to an empty house at 3:30 pm. I was absolutely shattered, laid on the bed and went straight to sleep. Karina woke me at 6:30 pm when she got in from work. I couldn't believe I'd been asleep for three hours. It was as if I'd only just closed my eyes. I was still fatigued and hit the Lemsip again.

Karina isn't one to let an ailment go unquestioned so started drilling me on why the Lemsips. Her concern was the cold feeling in my chest on a deep breath. I argued for some variant of a flu bug. Something I'd picked up from one of the conference delegates. Karina argued for some variant of something else. The phrase *let's keep an open mind* punctuated my attempts to downplay the situation. Coupled with *there's no harm in getting it checked out*. The approximate translation for these combined phrases is, *let's go and hang out with the shouty drunks for a few hours.*

I was so, adamantly against it. I was tired, fed up and felt bullied. I really had no desire to take part in the soap opera of A&E for four hours, only to be sent home and get to bed at 1 am. As a compromise, Karina suggested ringing 111. As a compromise on the compromise, I suggested that *she* phoned 111. I really couldn't be arsed to go through all the inevitable questions.

Clearly, I was firing on three cylinders. There was no way a 111 conversation about *me* was going to conclude without talking to *me*. *Me* really wasn't interested. When Karina passed the phone over, my tone was a blend of that used when accidentally answering a cold call selling cures for erectile dysfunction and discovering my car had been broken into and they'd wazzed on the driver's seat.

I answered all questions completely honestly and, in my mind, provided a tsunami of evidence as to why further discussion would be a waste of everyone's time. Towards what was becoming the end of the conversation, the extremely diligent and patient 111 nurse said, 'I think you know where this is going, don't you?'

And she was right, I did.

Within ten minutes Karina was driving me to our local A&E about five minutes away. I offered to drive but the 111 nurse had told Karina not to let me near the keys.

*Just to be on the safe side.*

# 4

## Dogs To The Left, Shite To The Right

*"The truth will set you free. But first it will piss you off."*
**Gloria Steinem**

My fears about a four-hour wait in A&E proved unfounded. It was barely half full, everyone was reasonably civilised, remaining in their seats to argue incoherently, and no one was being restrained by the local constabulary. It also appears if your triage story includes *something* in the chest, ongoing AF and a 111 nurse insisting on an immediate visit to A&E with someone else driving, it's the equivalent of Priority Boarding.

Within minutes, I was given a laminated sign reading 'ECG' and within a few minutes more I was in a consultation room having sticky pads attached to my body. There was the usual chitty-chatty stuff, and I was *that* patient going out of his way to apologise for wasting the nurse's time; explaining I was feeling absolutely fine and had only come in to keep the wife happy. I was pretty sure he was buying it until he said, 'Did you run here?'

Bizarre question. 'No of course not. Why?'

'Your heart rate is 155... but you're not even breathing heavy... or sweating.' He listened to my heart. 'Can you feel any fluttering in your chest?'

'Not at all.'

He went on to tell me my heart rhythm was very irregular, and I was in AF. He didn't seem very interested when I told him that was just something I lived with.

'Has it been like this all day?' he asked.

'No. It's been like this most of the year. And most of last year too. Come to think of it, most of the year before that as well. Like I say, I just live with it.' There was a slight beat as he looked at me for signs I was taking the piss.

Blood samples (always affectionately referred to as *bloods*) were taken followed by several pages of questions; the answers dutifully captured on yellow record forms. I then left that consultation room, but not back into the main waiting room. I was ushered through a different door into the *actual* A&E department. The place where it all happens. The engine room. The war-zone.

My spider senses were tingling. Heading further into the machine meant further engagement and from my experience a couple of years earlier when first diagnosed with AF, further engagement could eventually lead to someone asking, 'What do you want for breakfast?'

There were queues of patients on beds in the corridor; a cacophony of alarms going off; a constant tangle of high-volume medical chatter and staff, desperately trying to look like this really *was* the job they'd studied all those years for.

I was guided into what appeared to be an understairs cupboard and had a further grilling from a Doctor going over the same questions I'd already answered twice that evening. But this time it was pink sheets capturing the answers.

I felt we were going in circles and there was clearly nothing of concern going on with me. Certainly, nothing a sachet of yellow powder in a mug of hot water couldn't sort out. That was until the Doctor stood up, paused while ponderously nodding his head, then without warning, punched me in the solar plexus and whilst winded, he scythed my legs from under me, leaving me in a stunned, crumpled heap.

Metaphorically speaking. Although he might as well have done, when he said, 'I'm going to admit you. We're going to treat you as having had a minor heart attack.'

Karina and I were bewildered. At no point had we ever expected to hear those words. I had an immediate sense of 'not me' which came out as almost repeating his sentence. 'You think I've had a minor heart attack?!!'

'No, not necessarily. We simply can't be sure at this stage. But if we start treatment now, *if* you've had one then, the better the recovery you'll have. And if you *haven't* had one, then the medicine won't do you any harm,' and promptly gave me four aspirin to chew.

This guy seriously meant *start treatment now*.

Doc Bombshell disappeared to start the admission paperwork and left us to the aftermath of the hand grenade just lobbed our way. Despite having had treatments for AF, the words 'heart' and 'attack' felt as relevant to me as 'Olympic' and 'Champion'. Me? It was incomprehensible. Those words were for other folk.

But what had become very apparent was, I wasn't going home that night. We quickly diverted our focus onto the practical things: what to say to our teenage boys back at home; phoning Karina's sister to ask if she could stay at ours; telling Karina's Mum; letting work know. Of them all, telling the boys would be the hardest as I knew they'd worry the most. They were quite mature for their then ages of 17 and 14, but they simply didn't have enough life experience to see through the cautious nature of the NHS. At that age, 'keeping Dad in as a precaution for a potential mild heart attack, until tests can be carried out' translates as 'Dad's had a heart attack.'

I had an overwhelming desire *not* to share these developments with any of the people we urgently had to contact. I've never been a machismo sort of guy but I felt sharing this news implied a weakness – a frailty. It felt private and circumstances were forcing us to expose ourselves from that privacy. I resented my hand being forced to share this news. I suspect most of us feel that way about our own health. We don't necessarily want to share our bodily status with the rest of the world. Even though these people were far from *the rest of the world*, I was irritated we had to do it. And we really did have to do it. And quickly. Karina with a matter-of-factness and I with indignant resignation.

About an hour later, a nurse parked a bed outside our understairs cupboard and began cleaning the vinyl mattress with antiseptic wipes. She popped her head in and said, 'It'll be dry in no time – I'll just get some sheets.' Karina and I looked at each other. The symbolism and implication of a hospital bed being prepared for me, bore down heavily. I felt thousands of country miles from just six weeks earlier, almost skipping towards my private hospital bed, to the sound of bells & whistles.

Eventually, the time came to move into the war-zone proper. The nurse asked me to get onto the bed so the waiting porter could push me through. I told her that wouldn't be necessary. I'd walk and sit on it once we were there. Wherever *there* was.

'I don't think so. You're not walking anywhere,' the nurse replied in a tone that came out of nowhere. Two questions immediately came to mind:

'Just how fucked up am I?'

And

'When did I hand over control?'

Now, I don't want to fall into the cliches of describing this A&E department but there are reasons those cliches exist and I lived those reasons for the next few hours. For a start, my bed wasn't in an actual bay, it was between bays. A bit like Platform 9¾ but without the reward of the magical destination. This in itself was hardly an issue for me. A&E was clearly very busy and as everyone else's conditions had to be genuine, it was far more important they had proper bays, and not I. But the people in the bays immediately either side of me, kind of were an issue, because what Bay 9¾ did have, was a similarly unusual assortment of characters to Harry's departure platform.

To my right was a poor man having near permanent issues with his stoma bag. He vociferously shared this predicament with the nurses. A lot. He also shared it with his fellow patients, as his leaked stoma spores stealthily and silently shimmied through the air, settling on anything within 20 metres. Anything such as nasal hair. Specifically, my nasal hair.

To my left was a poor lady in arguably even greater distress. At least I think she was. It was difficult to tell because she only ever barked like a dog. Well, two or three dogs. Not the bark of happy dogs; pleased to see their returning owner or their leads being taken off a coat hook signalling imminent walkies. These were dogs that had spotted a burglar and were thinking *challenge accepted.*

Constant barking. Non-stop. In hindsight maybe what she really needed was a vet.

Sat on a chair outside the patient's toilet, was a frail-looking lady, possibly just entering her twelfth decade, flanked by two security guards. She was a little bit *shouty* and wasn't going out of her way to make friends, but we did wonder what she'd done to warrant two security guards. They made no attempt to stop her colourful running commentary on the department, so we could only guess she had previous here and the guards were choosing to pick their battles.

By comparison, I was well-behaved, polite, not believed to be in a critical situation, therefore not urgent and consequently, was very infrequently attended to. In this scenario, I was a non-needy outlier, which weirdly gave us some level of comfort. Funny how receiving virtually no customer service can be perceived as a positive experience.

An initial blood test had shown slightly elevated levels of troponin. (Time to don the white coat.) Troponin is a protein released into the bloodstream and indicates a likelihood that the heart has sustained some level of damage. A heart attack, even a mild one, would therefore result in raised troponin levels, hence the concern. Troponin levels can also be elevated for many other reasons, none of which really get you out of the frying pan whilst avoiding the fire, except possibly as a result of infection, strenuous exercise or severe stress.

I was injected into my abdomen with blood thinners, started on a high dose of beta-blockers and hooked up to a heart rate monitor. My heart rate fluctuated between 80 and 150, sometimes within seconds. This was my old friend AF playing its usual game, albeit at a more extreme level. AF doesn't always induce a permanently raised heart rate, hence my lack of breathlessness and sweating when the ECG was taken on arrival. Remember the morse code? It's a sort of shuffling beat interspersed with rapid hops, sometimes to the rate of what appears to be three beats per second. The monitors are so sensitive, they will pick this up and extrapolate that data to provide a 'per minute' rate. Hence a short run of 2-3 beats per second is recalculated as a heart rate of 150 bpm or above. If a heart rate was genuinely running at that level, in the absence of any cause for exertion, this really would be a troubling situation and would need to be got down, urgently.

Not that my heart rate didn't need to be reduced, it did. But the medics were aware as to why the rate *appeared* to be *so* high, which fed into their apparent lack of attentiveness. (That thing we kept regarding as a positive.) However, the monitor attached to me missed the memo about my AF being the mischievous trickster it was, as the alarm was in a near-permanent state of screech. It was an auditory retaliation to the olfactory assault from stoma man and thinking about it now, may have been a factor in reducing the lady next to me, to barking like Alsatians on roids.

At some time around 1 am, having sought permission, I was allowed to be disconnected from the heart rate monitor to walk to the toilet. That's another thing about going into hospital; the speed at which we cede authority to others; to strangers; to an institution, without ever really processing or questioning *why*. Only a few hours before, I'd been shocked when I realised I'd apparently had decision-making taken away from me, without ever having discussed, agreed to, or signed any terms of surrender.

Within those few hours, something had happened to me whereby I didn't even question the need to seek permission to use the toilet. Perhaps that was the point of the noisy alarm on the machine hooked up to me. Maybe it wasn't monitoring anything at all. Maybe the rapidly changing numbers were fabricated, and the constant screeching was designed to assault my senses and distort my view of reality, with the aim of securing compliance.

Or maybe the lack of sleep, both that night and after a very demanding four-day event was beginning to take its toll.

Having been to the toilet and got back on the bed, no one was in any rush to reconnect me to the screecher, which provided some relief – to everyone in the department. I had no drip, there were no more medicines administered, no further blood samples taken, and I was still sandwiched between two genuine bays. As time went on, we continued to interpret this lack of attention, not as a dereliction of duty but as a whole bunch of positive signs. Surely, they couldn't really think I'd had a heart attack? If it were that serious, they'd have kicked one of these malingerers out of a proper bay and put me in it. And I'd have been on loads of drugs; I'd be hooked up; on close watch and wouldn't be allowed out of bed. In line with the extensive medical training Karina and I both had. Which, as we've established, was none.

Whatever was going on, the situation would soon be rectified, normal service would be resumed, and life would return to something more familiar in the morning. In the meantime, we both needed to try and get some sleep, which miraculously, we somehow did. Karina on a plastic chair and me on my side, under a wafer-thin blanket and my coat, and with a pillow over my head to dampen the sound of stoma man, other people's alarms, and those bloody dogs.

Around 6 am, more blood was taken, more meds were given and observations or *obs* were taken. Medical folk abbreviate everything. It makes things sound a bit friendlier and if referring to quite severe situations or treatments, those severe situations or treatments don't sound quite so severe.

Within an impressively short period of time, a Doctor arrived and advised my trops (the friendly abbreviation for troponin levels) were down a little but were still slightly elevated. He came clean - they couldn't be sure whether a heart attack had taken place or not, but it was sensible to continue treating me as if it had, just as a precaution until further tests could be carried out. However, the immediate concern was getting my heart rate down. And, on that basis, he would be admitting me.

For the second time that night, we'd been blindsided by a hand grenade all too casually lobbed into a conversation.

We'd been reading positives into the runes all night, so to be told I wasn't going home, was absolutely gutting. We'd convinced ourselves that the worst-case scenario of a mild heart attack was just that. A worst-case scenario. But not the actual scenario. And although no one was saying that was the actual scenario, the outcome was the same as if it was the actual scenario, which was the removal of freedom and implication that all was not well with me.

Professor Hindsight would've told us that really, we shouldn't have expected anything other than this outcome. My diagnosis upon entry to A&E was a suspected mild heart attack and my heart rate was currently both the department's limbo *and* high-jump champion. Nothing had changed. Why on earth would they have sent me home? Now that really would have been poor customer service. My concern, my underlying fear was, in my experience of hospitals and medics over the previous two years, the more they keep looking for stuff, the more stuff they keep finding. And what's more, the path to successfully fixing that stuff never seemed to be a nice, neat, upward straight line.

# 5

## Impending Doom

*"Good judgement comes from experience.*
*And experience? Well, that comes from poor judgement."*
**Origin unknown**
**(But Dean Martin was a fan)**

Apart from tiredness, I felt totally fine by the time the porter arrived with a wheelchair to take me to the Acute Medical Unit (AMU in medi-speak). AMU is where they put you straight after A&E when they don't know where to put you or they do know where to put you, but there isn't a bed immediately available. Which is often.

My heart rate had dropped a little but was still high enough to be of concern. Just as when the bed had arrived at the understairs cupboard, seeing the wheelchair really jolted me. Knowing I was regarded as needing a wheelchair, was incongruous to me. My self-perception was being brutally challenged. Like even the oldest of folk, I still regarded myself as young(ish), fit(ish) and strong(ish). There was a dissonance between what I believed, and the reality being presented to me. What was unfolding seemed inaccurate and unfair to me. So, it must have been on that basis that my inner rebel tested the newly appointed authority in my life by asking, 'Is it ok if I walk there?'

The porter looked a bit surprised and asked if I felt OK, to which I confirmed, I did. This seemed to exhaust his extensive medical training and satisfy his curiosity and so I walked to AMU with the porter leading the way.

I'm not one of those people who threaten to sue because my car battery carried no *Do Not Drink the Acid* warning. But again, with hindsight, this was poor judgement on both our parts. Neither of us was qualified to make the decision allowing me to walk.

I'd been off my feet for 10+ hours by that point, so my heart hadn't really had a great deal to do beyond the bare minimum. But even that short walk required effort and by the time I'd got to my allocated bed, my heart rate was as high as it'd been on entry to A&E. Note to self: start taking this a bit more seriously. Note to the porter: don't make decisions above your pay grade.

I was directed to a bed by the window in a bay of six. I quite liked that position. It was bright and I only had the one neighbour to my right rather than being between two beds. This allowed for a bit more privacy and space but also meant I only had one person to ignore, rather than two. Little things like this, in institutions where you're all but stripped of control, can feel quite significant. These are the small wins, which I find, can make a huge difference in interpreting life experiences.

By early afternoon, my heart rate had come down a little but was still stubbornly high. A Doctor explained he was going to administer a drug that should bring the rate down quite quickly, but then started quite an intriguing conversation.

'Now, I have to tell you a lot of patients seem to experience quite an unusual side effect with this drug.' If this was supposed to calm me down, it was already having the opposite effect.

'What is it?' I nervously ask.

'Well, quite often as it's being injected, patients have quite a weird sensation.'

'What kind of sensation?' I really hoped it wasn't anything of a sexual nature.

'Well, we don't know why, but quite often they feel an over-whelming sense of impending doom... their faces look quite, well... terrified. They sometimes even try to get out of bed and run away... just for a few seconds... and then it goes away. But it's really effective at reducing heart rate.'

I was baffled. I was about to be injected with Class A drugs, legally. Karina's reaction was interesting.

'Can I film him when you inject it?' Which bizarrely, I was up for. Don't get me wrong, I was anxious about what an overwhelm-ing sense of impending doom felt like - but I was also really quite cu-rious how my face would take the news.

Then something *really* weird happened. Doctor Doom disap-peared and came back about five minutes later with a little tray con-taining the necessary vial, a syringe, plaster etc. He'd wiped my arm with the antiseptic swab when it became obvious that my heart rate had reduced. Considerably. All by itself.

The Doc smiled. 'That happens a lot too. For some reason, when we tell a patient about the side effect, it's quite common for their heart rate to drop, within minutes. No idea why.'

On the back of this sudden turn of events, Doc Doom decided not to administer the drug unless my heart rate went up again over the next hour. It didn't and as odd as it sounds, I felt a little robbed of my sudden, short-lived, overwhelming sense of impending doom. Karina felt a bit short-changed, too.

The reduction and stabilisation of my heart rate was very positive news but was by no means a get out of jail card. The medics still wanted to get to the bottom of the *was it/wasn't it* conundrum, which meant continued tests, an X-ray and more monitoring, so I wasn't allowed to get too comfy in AMU. Before I had a chance to tuck into the three-course evening meal, I was moved to the CCU (Cardiac Care Unit) and told some news that almost broke me.

I was told the only way to know for sure, whether I'd had a mild heart attack, was to carry out an Angiogram. (Where's my white coat?) In its simplest terms, an Angiogram is a procedure whereby a small incision is made in an artery in the wrist and a camera on a wire is fed through the arteries to the heart to inspect it for damaged tissue and blockages in vessels. All under local anaesthetic.

A heart attack is caused by a lack of oxygen to the heart muscle, (often caused by blocked blood vessels) which in turn can cause that muscle tissue to die. So, if a heart attack had taken place, even a minor one, the chances are, there would be evidence of damaged tissue.

Ok – that sounded straightforward, I thought. It probably requires a tad more skill than suggested by my description, but as medical procedures go, it sounded straightforward. They agreed it was a fairly routine procedure but unfortunately (and this was slightly galling), this fairly routine procedure was no longer carried out at my local hospital. I'd have to be taken to a much larger hospital, about 10 miles away. To some extent, this made sense. The larger hospital is a Centre of Cardiac Excellence, so I knew they'd be able to get to the bottom of it.

However, by then it was late on Thursday and there was no way it would be happening that day. The news continued to unfold. The following day was Good Friday, followed by Easter weekend and Easter Monday. I began to get a sinking sense of where this was going.

Unfortunately, the four-day Easter weekend meant reduced staff, reduced numbers of procedures and crucially, no Consultant* at that time, to request and sign off the procedure anyway. All in all, including the night I'd already spent in Bay 9¾, I was probably looking at the wrong end of a six-night stay.

Christ on a bike.

*Just for the sake of clarity, this was not Gordon, the Consultant I'd seen privately, as he didn't work in this hospital. Although at that point in time, it felt to me, that the Consultant employed by the hospital and allocated to me was also 'not working' – by choice.*

The initial galling had snowballed into a gut-full of galls; a gaggle of galls; a google of galls. Being told I had to stay in hospital for a further four days; not because I was in such bad shape, but because the NHS couldn't resource itself to provide what they themselves described as a *routine procedure* absolutely incensed me. I was particularly incensed about the lack of Consultant availability to even initiate the procedure. I had visions of this guy lapping up the weekend sunshine in St Andrews, playing golf, enjoying his power and authority to do just what the fuck he wanted, when he wanted, without any thought for other people's lives. Specifically - my life.

And not just any old weekend - Easter weekend. The weather forecast predicted belting weather over the four-day break – and so it proved. It was the hottest Easter weekend on record, and I love the sun. I cross the road to walk on the sunny side of the street. Karina laughs at me for moving my seat to face the sun and then bollocks me for not putting sun cream on. I love the heat on my face and body and after a six-month winter absence, the Easter sun had meant Easter fun. A fully deserved break in the middle of our crazy conference season. We'd planned to have the first BBQ of the year and that meant, friends coming round; a few beers; a few laughs and a cracking good time. Which couldn't have been further away from what I was looking at. I even took a photo from my hospital bed of what I was literally looking at: three bins, two hand sanitisers and a sink. Merry Eastmas.

But the biggest thing; the biggest upset for me was having to face the fact I'd now have to inform an ever-widening circle of people about the situation, and I'd also have to relay it in the present tense. If it were one of those, *oh you wouldn't believe what happened to me* type of stories, that would have been different. That would have been past tense, so whatever the issue had been, would have been resolved, because I, the storyteller, would be telling the tale within the context of *things have moved on*. But because of the Consultant golfing in St Andrews (he wasn't) and because NHS staff can't be arsed and either pull sickies or bunk off for Easter (they can and they hadn't), I was stuck in a hospital.

Whilst all the above was true (apart from the bits that aren't) and would feature in the wider sharing of my news, it was all padding around the central, crucial, and specific bit that I had to share, which was: I was in hospital because people far cleverer than I, were concerned that something quite serious might have happened to my heart.

I certainly felt fine, so I didn't want my family and close friends to worry, but there was something else. I didn't want people to think I was in some way damaged or weak, either. I can't imagine anyone (I was bothered about, at least) would have thought I was less of a person, less of whoever they saw as being *me*. And just as a reminder - I'm no bravado-boy, big on displays of testosterone. I'm no gobshite, peacock, alpha male presenting a perfect front. I'm big on mistakes! 'Embrace failure, Karl,' my Head of Sixth Form told me. (Read into that, what you will.) But until the previous couple of years, I'd never had cause to go to a hospital for myself. I suppose I'd had a quiet confidence in my latent fitness, and I've always been in reasonable shape. Cycling in the nearby hills had done wonders for my endurance.

Being in reasonable shape and having a pretty good level of fitness so far in life, meant that I'd believed I was scoring better than average in the *how's your health at 50* stakes. That was until the ablation six weeks prior. My self-belief had been challenged by the poor recovery from that, and now this. The disparity between my self-perception and the evidence I was being confronted with (which was actually not that much, but the inconclusive nature of which), felt very uncomfortable. Which meant, sharing my Easter status with friends and family, also felt uncomfortable. And I clearly couldn't hide it from them as I should have been seeing many of them over the gorgeously sunny Easter weekend.

If I could have gotten away with not telling anyone, I probably would have done. But that's not how the real world works. And it's not that nice on the people who care about us, either.

# 6

# Lost Weekend

*"You don't have to believe everything you think."*
**Erykah Badu**

It was baking on the ward that weekend. I was wearing cargo shorts and a t-shirt every day. Although I was hooked up to a heart rate monitor, it was a tiny thing so I could put it in a pocket and walk around. I watched masses of Netflix but was still bored. I couldn't help thinking of all the fun stuff everyone else was up to and the thought of having a few beers with our friends was never far from my mind. That really didn't help with my temperament.

To try and score time off quickly and give myself a sense of progress, I divided each of the four Easter days into units of morning, afternoon, and evening. With every unit that passed, I moved a little closer to getting out. So, by Saturday morning having a score of 4/12 felt pretty good. By Saturday at 6 pm it was 5/12... almost halfway there.

Karina came to visit every day and the boys came along on a couple of visits. Dad being in hospital with some sort of heart issue would have caused them some concern. Rightly or wrongly, we'd decided to leave out the *potential mild heart attack* bit and just go for the much woollier *pain in the chest*, as we still thought they'd just distil anything else down to *heart attack*. Besides, the consistent message coming from the white coats was that a heart attack was un-likely, but they needed the Angiogram results to make sure.

The first visit really reassured the boys; seeing me in summer clothes, looking normal, behaving normal, talking as normal and sharing my frustration just as any normal person would. In these cir-cumstances, *normal* is good, in the eyes of your kids.

On their second visit, they were probably as keen as me to leave. I can imagine the conversations that had taken place to even get them there. I got it and encouraged them all to get off and enjoy their weekends. Hospital visits can be wearisome at the best of times. I'm not sure when the best of times are for hospital visits, but when they coincide with a glorious four-day weekend, a CCU ward wouldn't make a Tripadvisor list.

My poor lads were struggling with the smell too. Hospitals have a smell about them – it's undeniable and everyone knows it. A sort of blend of disinfectant, embalming fluid, boiled cabbage, and bod-ily expulsions. When you visit, you expect it and prepare yourself for it and put up with it. That's just what you do and that's just the way hospitals smell.

Unless you're a teenage lad, in which case you bring it up every 30 seconds accompanied by facial contortions. By that time, the smell was wallpaper to me, which was a sure sign of sliding into being in-stitutionalised.

Good Friday morning didn't start well. Thursday night had been my first night in a ward bed and I was woken with a rude reminder I was no longer my own sovereign state. It'd been a noisy night on the ward so sleep had been more broken than not and ideally, I would have wanted to sleep until gone 9. Maybe even gone 11. At 7 am, I was physically jolted and cheerily shouted at to get out of bed by two nurses. Probably not shouted at, as such. Perhaps it was just the volume they used for those patients who had hearing aids but overlooked switching them on.

Apparently, they wanted to change the bedsheets. I mumbled something about, 'Don't worry - these are fine'. I felt quite cosy and anyway, I thought they'd appreciate having one less job to do. How they laughed as they explained that the sheets would be changed every morning.

*Every morning?!!*

I don't know how often you change your bedsheets but we don't change ours every sodding morning. Another point scored to the institution.

The Ward Sister came over, introduced herself and wrote a few details on a whiteboard on the wall, next to my bed. One of these details was my Consultant's name and with that, she brought good tidings. Apparently, he'd had a change of heart, cut short his golf trip in St Andrews and would be doing a ward round on Sunday. (Only part of this is true.) This was great news as I'd not expected to be seeing him until Tuesday. The Sister even went as far as to say, if he signed off the procedure, it could even happen on Monday.

Wow. My spirits lifted no end. This was a big win.

Sure – I'd still be bored for the next couple of days and would be missing out on the warmest Easter weekend in living memory, but the thought of being out on Monday made that easier to deal with. With a good wind, I may even get some of the afternoon and evening sat on our decking, soaking up some sun and enjoying a beer or two.

From a work point of view, I'd miss the setup of the next conference in Newcastle, but I'd travel a day later, early on Tuesday and pick up with the team. Normal service resumed with very little disruption. Result.

The whiteboard also had a section at the bottom that read: *what matters to me most*. The Sister asked what I wanted to put in this section. I wasn't entirely sure what the context was, so she offered some examples from other patients, such as: peace and quiet; independence; help with meals.

'To go home,' was my response and *being discharged* was duly written.

'A very understandable wish,' she said. Later that day, I went to the bathroom but rather than going straight back to my bunk, I thought I'd stretch my legs and walk to the end of the ward and back. As I did, at the risk of being nosey, I checked out my fellow inmates' whiteboards to see what mattered to them most.

Every whiteboard bore the same message. Peace and quiet, my arse. Every single patient dreamed of *being discharged* and why wouldn't they? Being in CCU isn't a lifestyle choice. But at least my pathway out was beginning to show itself. The end was in sight, and I'd soon be able to put this whole experience behind me.

True to his word, the Consultant did a ward round on the Sunday morning. He must have flown back from St Andrews the night before, as he looked pretty fresh and there was no hint of a pringle sweater or plus-fours. He wasn't the chattiest of fellows (probably got beat) but he made all the right noises. He confirmed he'd requested the Angiogram (win); he was very happy with my now much-stabilised heart rate; my blood pressure was fine; my ankles weren't swollen (not that they ever had been) and my $O^2$ levels had all been normal throughout my stay. He was also happy to hear that I'd been on my feet a fair bit (all wins). So, I thought this was a good time to ask him the direct question – did he think I'd had a mild heart attack?

'Mild heart attacks are always very difficult to accurately diagnose, hence the Angiogram. But looking at the evidence, if I was a betting man, which I'm not, I'd say no.'

Win. Big win. The man from Del Monte says no!

But he also reminded me, he couldn't, with 100% accuracy, say I hadn't had a mild heart attack. He went on to point out, one of the reasons I'd been kept in was that often a much larger, more serious heart attack could happen within a week of the mild one, which was something of a chilling thought. So, contrary to all evidence, it appeared I hadn't just been kept in because he'd wanted to play on a links course in the far north of Scotland. Which of course, he hadn't.

Despite this revelation, I slept well that night. 9/12 down and I might just catch the last two slots back at home. I'm pleased I got some decent sleep that night. It meant I didn't have to contemplate my own naivety when it came to managing my expectations of the NHS Beast.

I asked the Ward Sister (not Sister Whiteboard – a different one) quite early the following morning if she knew when I'd be going for the Angiogram. She explained that two things had to happen; The larger hospital had to provide them with a confirmed appointment and then an ambulance had to be found to take me there. She'd chase it up just as soon as she had finished a couple of things. That was about 8:30 am.

By 10:30 am she hadn't gotten back to me, and I was beginning to feel the impatience that only a patient can feel. My two slots at home were being eaten into, so I asked her again.

'Oh, I'm sorry – it slipped my mind.'

'Oh, that's ok, I completely understand. Don't worry – I'll work around you,' I absolutely didn't think and therefore didn't say. There was definitely some kind of non-verbal exchange though, as an attentive nurse suddenly piped up that she'd look into it straight away. Naturally, I appreciated the sudden expediency to her patient's cause. Thinking about it now though, I think they were getting to the point where they just wanted the bed back from the chippy bloke who seemed to be absolutely fine.

The nurse came back fairly quickly and far too merrily shared the news. 'No – it won't be today. They've had some emergencies over the weekend to deal with. It'll probably be tomorrow now.'

John Cleese's character, Brian Stimpson, famously said in Clockwise, 'I can take the despair – it's the hope I can't stand.' At that point in time, I was Brian Stimpson. I only wanted 2/12 of my Easter weekend. Even 1/12 would have done. Just a sliver of what everyone else had enjoyed and that would have been fine. But no. For reasons beyond I could reason, I was going nowhere. I was once again, gutted. All the wins seemingly dissolved away. Apart from everyone being pretty confident I hadn't had a heart attack. Funny how you can overlook the big wins when the little ones are crushed.

Tuesday 23rd brought better news – the other hospital could fit me in. The challenge then was securing an available ambulance to transfer me. Similar to the way I'd thought I was being helpful by suggesting my bedsheets didn't need to be changed, I told them not to worry about the ambulance. Karina could drive me over. It's only 25 minutes – 30 tops.

I was looked at as though I'd just confessed to eating one of my own kids. What followed was a mild motherly scolding from the Sister:

'You know why you're here don't you?' (This I took to be rhetorical.) 'And why you need the Angiogram?' (See above.) 'What if something was to happen to you on the way there?' (This I didn't take as rhetorical, so I took my chance.)

'Well, if something happened, we'd drive to the hospital, which is where we'd be going anyway.'

The look she gave me in the silence that followed, made me unsure as to whether Sisters had the authority to spit in patients' food. I decided to skip lunch anyway.

Apparently, I would most definitely be travelling in an ambulance. And guess what? None were available for the whole of Tuesday. It was a shocking day for trips and falls apparently. Perhaps everyone had still been wearing flip flops, clumsily, from the Easter heatwave I'd completely missed.

By then, like Brian Stimpson, I'd released my hope and was resigned to a Wednesday departure, Ironically, my resignation made the final day less of an endurance. Once the Angiogram was done, I'd go home and get myself sorted for the final two days of the week. I wouldn't make the conference in Newcastle, but we had a close friend's 50th birthday party the following weekend. The worst would soon be behind me, and sunlit days of Springtime freedom were around the corner.

# 7

## Lucky Man

*"Fate is like a strange, unpopular restaurant filled with odd little waiters who bring things you never asked for and don't always like."*
**Lemony Snicket**

24<sup>th</sup> April 2019 was going to be a great day. It was as sunny inside CCU as it was outside, the morning I was due to be transferred for my Angiogram. It felt that way to me anyway. And in the nicest possible way, the nurses seemed as keen for me to leave, as I was, to go. Not that I'd been a stroppy customer, but I clearly wasn't their average one. I'd spent pretty much the whole time fully clothed, walking about, needing virtually no attention, and yet was still taking a bed up. If there was an award for the *Low Maintenance Patient of the Year*... in the words of Brian Clough, 'I'm not saying I was the best candidate, but I was definitely in the top one.'

Leaving would be regarded as a win-win.

To the amazement of all, the ambulance arrived soon after breakfast. Given my imminent *Low Maintenance* nomination, I was more than a little surprised when the Paramedic wheeled the ambulance trolly-bed up next to me.

I somehow managed to head off my instinctive response of, 'You're shitting me, right?' and, once again attempted to be helpful. I advised the Paramedic I wouldn't be needing the trolley. I'd walk to the ambulance. We were on the ground floor and it was only parked 50 metres away.

Apparently, I wasn't being helpful at all and the Sister sided with him, the turncoat. She'd been comfortable enough with me walking around the ward for the last four days, yet suddenly I was deemed vulnerable. Vulnerable enough to be strapped to a gurney, and not just for the 50 metres. For the whole journey.

Negotiations followed and a compromise was agreed whereby I was allowed (allowed!) to sit in a wheelchair and be pushed to the ambulance. At that point, I'd sit in a chair in the ambulance rather than lay down. Another small win. They all count. I'm all for picking your battles but by then, I was picking them all.

It crossed my mind again though - just how bad a shape did these people think I was in? But then, I reflected whilst on the journey that it's their responsibility to be risk-averse, which to be fair, is where you want your medical support to be. Besides, I'd be in the Centre of Cardiac Excellence within no time and with a good wind, the procedure would be over quickly. I'd be home by early to mid-afternoon, almost a full week since I was talked into visiting A&E.

Upon arrival, I was taken straight to the Catheter (or Cath) Lab where the procedure would be taking place. Buoyed by the knowledge that I'd soon be out, it almost felt a little bit exciting for me to be there. What was it about me positively anticipating minorly invasive procedures? I must get that looked at. Which, in itself, would probably involve a procedure.

Once prepped, I settled down to read my book. The day was running like a Swiss clock. It wasn't even lunchtime so if anything, we were running ahead of my mental timings. I was very relaxed and almost content.

I didn't get to read for long before I was escorted through a different door, briefly along a corridor, through a double door and for the second time in my life, into an operating theatre. It really is quite an overwhelming sight for a patient. There were far more people this time and a lot more equipment. A huge screen was set up by a very narrow, raised bed, which I guessed, had my name on it.

There was a lot of politeness and a chap introduced himself as the Consultant who'd be carrying out the procedure. I was invited to lay down on the bed, which felt odd as it was too narrow for my arms, but then supports were slid in, which felt much better. A rather pleasant surprise was a heated blanket being placed over me by a person unseen. The support for my right arm was extended out to 45 degrees from my side; clearly, this was going to be the point of entry.

All this time, the Consultant had been talking to me, asking about my original symptoms, asking about my job. I sensed it was more chit-chat than fact gathering. I certainly hoped so. It'd be nice to think he'd at least skim-read my notes before strapping me onto the bed and shoving an unbent wire coat hanger through my slit wrist.

Within seconds, a local anaesthetic was injected into my right wrist and the procedure was underway. I can honestly say I didn't feel a thing. It took about 45 minutes, and I was occasionally asked if I was OK (which I was). I felt unusually calm and relaxed. Maybe there was some other additive in that anaesthetic.

There was constant chatter throughout this time. I'd initially tried to follow what was being said, to see if I could pick up on anything. They were using English words, but I had no idea what they meant. Measurements and percentages were shared but the team appeared to use vocabulary unique to those four walls. I occasionally looked at the huge screen... Wow – that was my heart! Or some part of it. It could have been a scan of the inside of an Egyptian mummy for all I knew. There was nothing I could decipher and no evidence I was capable of interpreting. As such, it'd been an uneventful, stress-free, and painless procedure. The Consultant confirmed completion, by concluding with, 'Right – all finished.'

After all the waiting, it was finally, finally, over and in the words of Messrs Simon & Garfunkel, I'd soon be *homeward bound*. My spirits were high.

The Consultant came round to my left-hand side whilst someone was applying a dressing to my right wrist. Naturally, I asked if he could tell if I'd had a heart attack.

'Well, I have good news. I can see no damaged tissue and no evidence of a heart attack so have to conclude that no, you didn't. It could well have been a viral bug which is why you were a bit achy generally and your lungs felt sore when you took a big breath. We can't know for certain what it was, but there's definitely no tissue damage.'

Confirmation at last! A big win. Finally, firm evidence that the worst hadn't happened. I can't tell you the bubble of elation and relief I could feel welling up inside me and how much I was looking forward to sharing the news with Karina. Not that I'd been worried but there was always inevitably a little bit of doubt as, far too often for my liking, I'd been treated as though I was as fragile as eggshells. How wrong they had been.

'However...'

Only one word, but it was like a seat belt locking in an emergency stop.

'Look mate, I've already got the fireworks out of the box – don't give me "*however*"'... I wanted to say.

'Completely by chance, we discovered one of the three main arteries on your heart is approximately 90% blocked. Usually, to treat this, we'd insert a small mesh tube called a stent, which would go into the blocked area. We'd then inflate a small balloon which presses the stent against the artery walls, allowing the blood to flow freely again.'

I got that this wasn't great news, but he'd just described the solution and he appeared to be asking for consent. 'OK – let's crack on then,' I offered.

A gentle smile. 'That's what we'd *usually* do and usually, we'd do it now - following on from the Angiogram. But the length of this blockage is juuuuuu-st on the limits of what a stent can handle...' He made a slowly increasing gap between his thumb and forefinger as he drew out the word *just* and followed up with, 'So I'm going to book you in for a heart bypass – it should be early next week, I'd imagine.'

And there it is: *the fuckening.*

Just when your day is going too well, and you don't trust it; sensing that some shit will eventually go down.

Being told this information just needs to hang in the air a while. He said it as nonchalantly as if asking how I was fixed for a dental appointment next Tuesday. The juxtaposition between content and delivery couldn't have been greater but both rounded on me as a single uppercut. My Fight-Flight-Freeze survival instincts froze on freeze.

I'd love to be able to recount in detail, the conversation that immediately followed, but I honestly can't remember a thing. I assume I replied. My Mum would've been very disappointed with my manners if I'd just stopped my half of a conversation and had left the other person hanging. But I have no idea which words were exchanged or in what order, immediately after this bombshell was so passively delivered. The week before I'd been on Lemsips. Now I was having a heart bypass. How did I get from one to the other?

At that point, I didn't even really understand what a heart bypass was. My Mum had a triple bypass about 18 years earlier, but my understanding of what that meant in detail, was scant beyond, *here's your heart mate and here's the shiny new dual carriageway bypassing it.* The thoughts and emotions came thick and fast, like a tsunami swallowing up my old reality and immediately creating a new landscape, much messier than the first.

*Me?* was a very loud and clear thought.

*Me? I was going to have a heart bypass?*

There was a complete disconnect between me the person, me – how I was feeling, me the 50-year-old... and this old person's operation. That was the biggie.

He was talking about something which happened to old people. *OLD* people. I wasn't old. This can't be right. Was my heart in the same condition as someone in their 70s or 80s? Was I that broken? I had no sense of being that broken. Only a few minutes before, I was fully expecting a clean bill of health (except for the AF) and had been looking forward to going to a friend's 50th at the weekend. A chance to catch up on the four-day funfest I'd missed, the previous weekend. Now it appeared I had something else to look forward to. An alternative future. Perhaps a short future too, given that a rather crucial part of my body was apparently already in its 80s.

It wasn't just the age-inappropriateness of the operation that hit me, it was also the scale. Although I was yet to fully understand exactly what a heart bypass entailed, I knew it was a bit more than having an ingrowing toenail sorted out. I knew it was a big operation. A long operation. A serious operation. The kind where things don't always go to plan. The game in which I'd found myself an unwilling player had just stepped up several levels.

Only a few days prior, I'd been knocked off my feet when the possibility of a mild heart attack had been floated. How I longed for a return to those days of jest and jape. That rose-tinted recent past, when benign words like 'possible' and 'mild' were used in the context of my health. How we'd all laughed when they'd been banded around.

But now - the Jumanji drums were pounding louder than ever and the lack of control I felt was overwhelming.

Possibly words tumbled out of my mouth. Or maybe I can't recall what I said because I didn't say anything. Perhaps I just stared at him blankly, like a man buffering. Whatever my response, the Consultant had been around long enough to recognise a man in shock. He suddenly adopted a far more softened, empathetic tone. My memory re-engages with him following me into the Recovery Bay. As I was parked up with other Jumanji players, he left me with his parting comments.

'I won't be operating on you - that's not my speciality but please try and remember these two things: it won't feel like it yet, but this is amazingly good news. We now know about this blockage and can do something about it. You've been walking around with a ticking time bomb inside you – and with a blockage of 90%, there's not much time left on the fuse. Thousands of people are walking around with them and sadly, only their relatives will ever get to know they had them. Secondly, this is a Centre of Excellence for cardiology. You're in one of the best places in the UK for this operation, with the best surgeons and facilities. You're actually a very lucky man.'

I was left in my own company for a while, whilst the admin was started for my admission to hospital for the second time within a week. It was my first opportunity to begin to process how events had unfolded over the previous few minutes.

*Lucky.*

It's a curious word. We usually associate it with winning something, gaining something, being better off for having something; especially when either the odds were stacked against us or the outcome had been random. I'd never have thought that needing a major operation could be classed as *lucky*. But in my shocked state, I even surprised myself. I attached my emotions to the life raft of the parting words of the Cardiologist.

I had a hitherto undetected, life-threatening problem. The problem had been discovered. The skills and technology were available to rectify the problem. Rectification would take place the following week.

What were my options? If I didn't have this operation or more to the point if I'd remained unaware as to what was going on inside my chest, what would happen to me?

*Not much time left of the fuse.*

You didn't have to be a Bletchley Park codebreaker to work that one out. Completely contrary to how I'd ever imagined I would've reacted to such news, I latched on to *lucky*.

I realised the truth very quickly. I genuinely was *winning something; gaining something; better off for having something...* the opportunity to stay alive. Is there a bigger prize?

So, yes – I was indeed a lucky man. A very lucky man. Lucky that Karina had forced the 111 call to happen, which led to the trip to A&E. It was then that it dawned on me. Karina had just saved my life.

Don't get me wrong, I wasn't getting the fireworks back out of the box again, but I saw this as a win. Heavily disguised and somewhat blurred around the edges, sure. But buried in there somewhere, was a feeling that this, terrible, distressing news, was a positive thing.

If receiving the news had been a shock, albeit one I was already trying to flip; worse than receiving the news, was the realisation that I now had to share it with the rest of my world.

Starting with Karina.

# 8

## Little Lord Fauntleroy

*"Happiness can be found, even in the darkest of times,*
*if one only remembers to turn on the light."*
**Albus Dumbledore**

A kindly nurse had gone to collect my belongings from the locker in the Cath Lab as, in my previous world, I would've been heading back there before skipping out of the hospital and back to my normal, bypass-free, everyday life. That world was long gone. Someone had switched points on the train track of my life, and I was now on a different route. The scenery would be unusual for a while and the journey not quite what I'd ever expected. But hopefully, the general direction of travel would remain roughly the same.

My bag was laid on my bed. I retrieved my phone and made the dreaded call. And I *was* dreading it. The content would be difficult, but more so for how it would impact Karina.

I've heard it said that often, people who have been diagnosed with cancer find it harder and more painful, having to tell their close family and friends, than when they received the news themselves. I can understand that sentiment. At that point, I was far more concerned about how Karina and the boys would feel, rather than what I would ultimately be going through.

Karina was at work, waiting for my call, ready to collect me whenever I phoned. I pressed Karina's speed dial. The phone rang. What was I going to say? What *was* I going to say?

Karina answered and after a few seconds of pleasantries I said, 'Well... it's not the result we were hoping for...'

Once again, I'm not sure of the exact conversation, but Karina tells me I was very calm, talked her through the news and what had happened to get there. As you'd expect, there were more questions than answers but our crash course in cardiac medical training hadn't fully started. That would change over the coming weeks.

After the phone call a male nurse was completing some admission admin and said, 'So, you're staying with us for a cabbage?'

I wasn't sure if I'd misheard but I went along with it. 'I hope not, I hate cabbage.'

He apologised for talking in acronyms and explained that a cabbage was in fact a CABG – a Coronary Artery Bypass Graft. A heart bypass to you and me, but to medical folk, it's a CABG (pronounced cabbage – hence my confusion). Yet more abbreviations and my cardiac medical training was underway.

So, yes, yes, I would be joining them for a CABG, next week apparently. I 'fessed that apart from the clue in the name, I didn't really know much about the procedure.

At this point, his enthusiasm dial turned sharply upwards. 'Obviously, the first thing they have to do is crack your sternum and then pull your ribcage open...' I was pleased I hadn't met this particular nurse before my phone call with Karina. I'm not sure I would have sold the concept of being *lucky*, quite so convincingly.

I was eventually wheeled to a cardio-thoracic ward, where Karina was waiting for me at the entrance, such was the time it took to process the paperwork and secure a bed.

I was taken to the end bay in the ward. This was a result as it meant no passing traffic and so probably a bit less noise. And I was in an end bed again, which, as you now know, is my preferred position, so no complaints there.

Well, I wasn't complaining at that point at least. After the first few nights though, I most definitely *was* complaining. Not in an out-loud, to anyone-who-could-do-something-about-it, sort of way. More in a keep-my-mouth-shut-unless-it-was-to-Karina, sort of way. My dissatisfaction was borne out of the Nurses' Station being right next to this end bay. As anyone who has spent time as an inpatient knows, with the Nurses' Station comes 24-hour lights being on, 24-hour alarms, 24-hour conversations and 24-hours of Celebrations being unwrapped. Within a few days, I'd engineered a work-around and was wearing an eye mask and earplugs when I settled down at night, which improved the length and quality of my sleep no end. Although, during those early days, because of this attempt at nocturnal sensory deprivation, I'm pretty sure I was labelled *the flighty new posh wanker on the block* by my fellow Jumanji players. I didn't care though. The earplugs also helped reduce the dark thoughts which accompanied middle-of-night emergencies taking place, because I heard fewer of them. My first left-hand neighbour required major medical attention in the middle of my second night. I never saw him again. That kind of stuff can sit heavy on your mind.

There were also middle-of-night admissions which seemingly unfolded at full daytime volume, which couldn't be ignored. One memorable nocturnal admission was Terry. Now Terry clearly enjoyed a tipple and on that particular night, he must have been tippling like it was 1999. At some point, the tippling had become too much for his svelte-like 28 stone body because he was brought in with breathing difficulties, AF, and chest pain. The reason I know he weighed 28 stone was that he shared that nugget with us at about 2 am. Us and the surrounding seven postcodes.

A nurse was trying to extract information and reason with him. Terry was clearly a regular as she was asking him if his home life had improved. He confirmed that it had. His new flat was nearer his local pub.

It was wrong of me, I know, but I was sniggering under my sheets. It wasn't a cruel sense of schadenfreude. It was just the sheer comedy value of the sketch taking place opposite me. It got better. The nurse then asked, 'Are you still smoking Terry?'

'Yes.'

'How many a day, roughly?'

'It depends.'

'OK, what does it depend on?'

'It's usually about 60 a day unless I've got a date that night... then it's only about 40. Cos I don't want my breath to smell.'

Nurses are trained not to laugh out loud at patients, so I did it for her. A good ol' LOL. I don't think that did me any favours in the early days either. It transpired that the pain in Terry's chest had been a mild heart attack, although his Doctors were at a loss to explain why it hadn't been a full-on, end of the line, heart attack. So, Terry joined me as a fellow member of the *Lucky Club*. He and I in a shared life situation. Dear God.

So, there I was, having recently celebrated my 50th birthday, holed up in a cardio-thoracic ward, waiting for a CABG. I've already briefly touched on it, but one of the most incongruous things for me was that this shouldn't be happening to someone of my age. I'd thought this was an older person's problem. But looking around the ward, this clearly wasn't the case. Sure, there were plenty of guys in there older than me; some in their 70s, 80s and beyond. But there were dozens in their 50s and 60s. Some were even much younger.

I'd always known on some level; middle-aged blokes could be prone to heart issues. But not this middle-aged bloke. This middle-aged bloke was fit and healthy. Or so I'd thought. This was reality brought into sharp focus. Nearly half the ward appeared to be within five years either side of my age.

Many patients were very frail and visibly poorly. Not all were in for the CABG treatment. Some were having second bypasses. Others were having valve replacements. Some had had heart attacks; many were in for a combination of these issues and some were due to co-morbidities just playing havoc on their cardiovascular system in general.

But given how I physically felt, my mobility, and my independent capability, looking at the condition of most of my fellow roomies, regardless of their age, I still felt so out of place. I was a goat amongst a flock of sheep. A horse within a herd of zebras. A Cornish Pasty amongst a tray of Steak Bakes.

I'd love to be able to report that I'd had the selfless, moral and humane disposition *not* to ask, 'Why me?' but that simply wasn't the case. Hell no. In fact, it was the complete opposite. I asked myself that question repeatedly. The fair and honest response should have been, 'Why not me?' The grown-up inside me should really have pointed out that I'd no more right to avoid this sort of thing, than the next person. But I wasn't that strong, or selfless. I felt that I'd been *wronged* to be in that situation. That it wasn't fair.

For a start, I could list half a dozen people who should have been ahead of me in the queue for this sort of shit. Fast food connoisseurs, heavy smokers, people stressed beyond measure – combinations of all three. Surely, they should've been more likely than me, to have ended up in that bed, in that ward, at that time.

For a while, I even harboured something close to resentment at being fast-tracked ahead of those people. Thinking about them began to piss me off. I know. Probably not my finest hour in terms of being at one with humanity. But come on, I had a lot of time on my hands and when you're surrounded by a scene the Ghost of Christmas Yet To Come might conjure up, misplaced self-pity comes easy.

I came to realise though; it was a waste of energy thinking like that. What does it change? But also, it eventually sunk in that, it said more about me than them. Why should someone be ahead of me in the queue just because they're more stressed or weigh more? Besides, for all anyone knew, they may well be in the same queue as me but just hadn't been lucky enough to discover it.

Eventually, the *why me and not them* thinking evolved into just some degree of surprise that it was happening to *me*. More of a, 'Who would have thought it?' And then ultimately, I settled on full acceptance of my new reality. I know this because at some point I began to use the phrase, 'We are, where we are'. And where we were, was in the process of learning the transition into patient life.

At some point in the morning, a menu card would be dropped on my table, and I'd select my lunch and evening meal, both of which had three courses. I'm not going to knock the quality of hospital food. It was generally pretty good, and three options were offered. But one was a sandwich, and one was a salad, so if you wanted a *meal* meal, then it was always the third choice – no matter what it was. If I were to offer a Google review though, the portion sizes were a little on the small size. But then an octogenarian's stomach is probably not the size it once was.

Now, back in the days when I was oblivious to my shortened fuse, there's no way I'd have been tucking into a three-course lunch and dinner - every day of the week. But it didn't stop there. Compared to my acutely poorly or post-operative roomies, I was an Olympic athlete. I was allowed to wander the hospital corridors in my shorts and t-shirt, ostensibly keeping mobile but mostly trying to manage the boredom. Eventually, I'd find myself in front of the hospital M&S Foodshop, picking up snacks and meal deals to fill the gaps between mealtimes whilst watching Netflix.

There were notices dotted around the wards and corridors informing patients and visitors that for every week a patient spent on a hospital bed, they lost 10% of their muscle mass. So, it was important to encourage patients out of their beds and to eat as much as possible. I took this to heart and even early on, began to gain weight. Who puts on weight in hospital? And to be honest, I was probably already carrying a bit of timber.

Given I was nowhere near as active in hospital as in civilian life, it's a wonder why I consumed so much. Possibly because it was there, and it was just something to do (boredom management is a massive part of hospital life). But also, there must have been some subconscious machinations going on. Some evolutionary, self-preservation drive, sensing that in a few days, I'd be going through something majorly traumatic and I'd need my strength and reserves.

I'm quite a sociable person, but I wasn't keen on having too many visitors. Partly because I really couldn't be arsed repeating all the same updates and answering the same questions. But there were other, more personal reasons. I didn't want to be on show, and I didn't want to feel my situation was currency for gossip. That's probably being very unkind to the people who might have visited. If they'd been bothered enough to make the time to visit, it would've been for genuine reasons of concern. Let's face it, everyone is busy enough without fitting in time for a hospital visit.

Also, I still had this sense of, 'What does this say about me?' Was I weaker by needing this operation? Was I perceived as being weaker? Less of a person than I was before? Was I more vulnerable? If I wasn't sure how I'd answer these questions, what would visitors be thinking? Or maybe, the more people visited, the more real this situation became, and subconsciously, I was still struggling to accept it was really happening.

I'm not fully sure of the reasons. I just know I wasn't keen on masses of visitors. Mostly it was Karina, occasionally with the boys, Karina's sister, Sarah and her husband, my brother-in-law, Justin. Karina's Mum visited once or twice and a few mates dropped by, but Karina was there every day. In hindsight, me not putting the welcome mat out for visitors probably put more pressure on Karina, to fill those long afternoon and evening hours with conversation, news, and gossip. Ordinarily, we wouldn't have spent that long every day in conversation. Routines like our day jobs and one of us watching Love Island would get in the way.

Bizarre as it sounds, I was pleased the boys didn't visit too often. They knew Dad was OK, and they had their own lives. George had A levels to be revising for, so I really didn't want him distracted. Ben also had school exams looming. Neither of them seemed to be overly concerned (beyond the smell) but they're both deeper thinkers than they let on, so I suspected they may be more concerned than they looked.

Around 9 pm, the meds were dished out. I was on aspirin and a blood thinner, but I must have been seriously fucked up because the blood-thinning injections kept on coming. I dreaded them. I dreaded them like a wuss.

I might have been reading or watching Netflix on the iPad, but I'd keep stealing glances, looking at the nurse with the meds trolley. How many more to me? How long to go? Then she'd get to me and be all chatty, in that nursey way. She'd sort out my meds and put them in that little paper cup for me to take afterwards. After what? After she'd prepared the needle.

I've built this up as if she were about to carry out an epidural. But then, I am that wuss. The truth is, there wasn't that much to prepare. They were the tiniest, pre-loaded syringes, with quite small needles really. Sometimes the skin pinch hurt more than the needle. There was a little 'pop' as it hit the skin. As the liquid went in, it felt cold and a bit sore but was over in seconds. There was always a bruise at every puncture site which lasted a few days, so over time, my abdomen (I'd struggle to keep a straight face if I said 'abs') looked like I'd been beaten with a bar.

More reading, Netflix, or texting night-nights; a quick trip to the loo and that was the day done. And then it started all over again.

It's honestly astonishing how quickly a seemingly independent and individual human being can become institutionalised. And not just institutionalised – willingly so. Still, as I've said before, it wasn't a lifestyle choice to be in there. And, when you considered that every member of staff who crossed my path was somehow contributing to trying to improve the quality of my life, there was little point in pushing back too hard about having clean sheets every day.

# 9

# Between A Rock And A Comfy Chair

*"I'm not telling you it's going to be easy,*
*I'm telling you it's going to be worth it."*
**Art Williams**

Within a few days of admission, I was visited by Dr A - Gordon, who had carried out my ablation. Whilst he had a private clinic, like many Consultants, he still spent most of his time working in the NHS. And with the hospital being a Centre of Cardiac Excellence, where else would he be based?

He wasn't my appointed Cardiologist, but he had declared an interest in my case, so was able to provide others with background information. It was fantastic to see a friendly face, someone who knew my story and would have my back.

Even as I type those words, they sound terribly unfair as everyone had been fantastic by that point. There were no unfriendly faces and I never suspected that anyone didn't have my back. But it was reassuring to have *my man* on the team.

That said, having steeled myself for a heart bypass – a CABG, no less, Gordon rather threw a medical spanner in the works. He advised they hadn't totally ruled out stenting the blockage after all, so a bypass wasn't a given. The thought of the bypass being bypassed was very appealing. Very appealing indeed. This was like having a serious and lengthy prison sentence commuted to *tidy up your bedroom*. I was elated at the possibility. Good news at last. Finally, something was beginning to go right. Maybe a corner was being turned and this would all be over quicker than I'd imagined.

My case was being discussed at a Multidisciplinary Team (MDT) meeting and a decision would be made as to which route was best for me. This sounded straightforward. Experts discussing factual things, sharing information, and coming to a consensus based on solid scientific knowledge. Surely this would be black-and-white territory.

Gordon went on to explain a lot had to be taken into consideration. They had to weigh up what they regarded as the best long-term outcome for me, against the invasiveness of different solutions. Hello – shades of grey seemed to be returning.

Let's just take a brief time-out here. To understand what was being discussed, we could probably do with a quick review of some basic cardiac physiology. Although I'm now a lay expert, at that stage, my O' Level Biology was a little rusty, so I'd imagine yours may be too.

The heart doesn't *just* pump blood around the body, it also needs a blood supply of its own, delivered through a series of many arteries. Three of them can be classed as the main arteries. Even these main three aren't all equal. Mr Big is the Left Anterior Descending artery (you guessed it, there's an abbreviation), the LAD artery.

The LAD feeds blood to the whole front wall of the heart, which is much more muscle than either of the other two major coronary arteries. As such, a narrowing or blockage in this artery is far more serious than narrowing or a blockage in any of the others.

In my case, it was the LAD becoming blocked. A blockage is a build-up of plaque that sticks to the artery walls and itself, causing the space through which blood can flow, to become narrower and narrower. This means that less and less oxygen is delivered to the heart, which can lead to a heart attack and ultimately death. I was hoping for alternative outcomes.

As I say, although I won't be opening up a private clinic anytime soon, I can now more than hold my own in a two-minute cardio conversation with a bloke in the pub. Let's get back to the ward.

So, there was a debate as to whether the CABG would be a more productive procedure or if the less invasive balloon Angioplasty with stenting, would do the job just fine.

I expressed a lot of confusion as I'd understood the stenting opportunity had been rejected at the time of the Angiogram. After review apparently, it was now considered stenting wasn't off the table. This was music to my ears. The least invasive, the better, as far as I was concerned. If I could avoid having my sternum cracked, my ribs pulled apart, being put on a heart/lung machine whilst the surgeons sliced through my flesh and arteries, I somehow felt, that would be a good thing.

There was also the subtext of the stenting route. The subliminal message that, if all the cracking and cutting didn't have to happen, then whatever was wrong with me, wasn't that bad after all. That I wasn't the broken-down shadow of the person I'd been before because - hey, just a tiny cut in the wrist and I'd be out the same day. Fixed.

But for the first time, the conversation opened up, and my trusted Cardiologist explained how effective the different routes would be, over time.

Once again, I apply the caveat that the following is based on what I recall being told about various procedures. Please don't use this information as a source for making decisions about yourself or your loved ones. And certainly not as a source for cramming for final medical exams.

Stenting, it appears, can be successful for between 5-10 years. Sometimes a lot longer, but it's likely that further work would be required. The nature of the stent can also mean that plaque sometimes attaches to its mesh, resulting in further narrowing. The stent can also only provide support for that section of the artery. The same artery could still become narrowed, further up or downstream from the stent, although further stents could be added.

A CABG would provide a longer-term solution – for decades or even up to the end of life were mentioned. Especially if an internal artery (the Mammary Artery) was used, rather than having to harvest veins from the legs. 'End of life' is a kind of arbitrary term but I was on the lookout for positive vibes, so I took that to mean in the 70-80-90 years region. As opposed to shortly after the operation, whereupon complications would cause a somewhat early conclusion to my time on planet Earth.

But apparently, there were other benefits to open-heart surgery too. Woo-hoo! Would I wake up with superpowers or a timeshare in Monaco?

No. The other benefits were that, as the heart would be right there in front of the surgeons, additional work could be carried out which would result in a more efficient cardiac performance once everything was put back under the bonnet. 'Such as?' you're probably thinking, which is why I asked, 'Such as?'

Remember that leaky Mitral Valve? The MDT saw open heart surgery as an opportunity to repair it. Once again Gordon stressed that ordinarily, they wouldn't have considered going to the lengths of surgery for a valve in this condition, as the leakage was only categorised as mild. But the repair would only add about 45 mins onto the operation and cardiac performance could be massively increased.

It was also suggested that further work could be carried out to address my AF. In fact, possibly even to nail it once and for all.

Gordon then hit me with his best sales line. 'You're young and strong, you're otherwise healthy, you haven't got any other issues like diabetes or lung problems – this might be an opportunity to repair a lot and secure a much more predictable future.'

And obviously, he delivered it with the calm, complete authority of a 12$^{th}$ Dan Jedi Knight, applying a tried and tested mind trick.

Only he wasn't. He wasn't selling anything. He wasn't pushing anything. But for the first time since this whole adventure had started, I felt I was being given information in the round. I felt I had some clarity on the nature of the issue and had learned, as with so many things in life, there are many solutions or even combinations of solutions, that could apply to any given problem.

Within a matter of minutes, I'd gone from totally accepting I was having a heart bypass to hang on, no need for all that cracking and slicing and slow painful recovery; back to maybe there was something in the old adage, *no pain, no gain* after all.

I had much to discuss with Karina and the MDT crew would be coming up with their decision imminently. Meanwhile, so as not to lose any time, all the pre bypass tests and preparations would continue, anyway. I felt like a man between a rock and a very comfy chair but was surprised to find myself so warmly eyeing up the rock.

# 10

# The Vacuum

*"If you think adventure is dangerous, try routine. It's lethal."*
**Paulo Coelho**

Being an inpatient for a significant time creates a vacuum, which used to be filled with so much everyday stuff – not least, work. There was never enough time in the day to get everything done. A spell in hospital is the hyper-opposite. There's so much time and so little to fill it. Hence my pre-occupation with eating. Not to mention all the clutter people send you on the phone and bring in: puzzles, books, newspapers, magazines, games, sweets, more food, weird WhatsApp films, memes and depending on who it was from, even weirder WhatsApp films. They know who they are.

But because of the peculiar distortion of the space-time continuum within hospitals (this has been proven by physicists, possibly), periods of time can sometimes appear exaggerated. Periods such as waiting for something to take place. Like a test of some sort.

Sometimes it genuinely seems like nothing is happening. But that can't be true. Medical teams will be working as fast as they are able to process requests. Us patients rarely consider that. We also don't consider the relativity of our own urgency versus that of others. Was I urgent? Hell yes – there wasn't much fuse left. But were there others with even less fuse? Or even fuse-less patients? Definitely, probably. (Oasis – you can have that as the title for your reunion album.)

Patients approach a hospital stay as a Black Ops Mission: they want to go in, get the job done asap and get out with no casualties. Especially themselves. The reality is a hospital is a collaboration of people, skills, specialities, resources, systems and checks & balances. It's an organism continually adapting to the needs of the people already inside the building as well as those being wheeled through the front door 24/7. I'm not surprised it doesn't run to a bus timetable. But then again, neither do buses.

I could have filled almost all of that time lag, working. Karina had often referred to me as a workaholic. I may be wrong, but I understood a workaholic to be someone who enjoyed working all hours. That wasn't me. It's just that there was always so much that needed doing in a small business.

Don't get me wrong, I used to really enjoy the whole event management game but, in the years prior, I'd felt more pressure and less enjoyment. Whether it was team issues or client demands, the more we provided, the less grateful some people became. Not everyone, obviously. A minority, but enough to take the edge off. Many clients, we loved and most staff over the years were incredible. But some of both had been testing. Toxic even. I'm sure staff and clients would be horrified to hear this. In some respects, it's human nature to take what was once was very much appreciated, as the norm, and so demand even more to be wowed. In other respects, some people are just incredibly selfish human beings.

This had been a significant factor in initiating the MBO conversation. However, I was also acutely aware that whatever was happening inside my chest, was significant enough to demand my full effort in resolving it. So as early as my first full day of being in this second hospital, I contacted my deputy to say I would be stepping back from Assured Events for a while, as I couldn't afford to give it any headspace or energy.

This was a big move for me. I'd never done it before, not even on holiday. As with many small business owners, I had tight control over access to finances and had the last say on recruitment and employee remuneration. Only the bookkeeper and I had access to the company bank accounts. I was totally serious about standing back because for the first time ever, I gave my deputy the passwords and access codes to the banking fob. She could now see all our accounts and access funds at will. I also handed over all aspects of employee management including making decisions on hiring, firing (if necessary), pay rises and awarding days in lieu. It was a huge amount of extra responsibility, if not actually masses more work. I offset the guilt for the additional responsibility by thinking she'd be taking on the role soon anyway, once she became the business owner.

I just knew if I didn't let go, it would hurt me. Badly. I was hardwired to keep control of the business and continue working in and on it. But I had to ask myself the question: is deciding to hold on, helpful to me, my family, our world, or would it be unhelpful? My inner voice had responded very quickly.

Although filling time was the perpetual challenge, as I've already alluded, I didn't want to be swamped by visitors for the full allowance. That said, visitors beyond Karina were most definitely welcome; it was just a question of when and for how long.

One pal talked his way in at 8 am on a Saturday morning. He'd told the nurses he was flying through from Singapore to the States with a brief stopover at the nearby Airport and this was his only chance to get a 15-minute visit in. Truth was, he was heading off to a golf day and the hospital was on the way. He left me a Times newspaper, and two magazines: one on superyachts and the other on vintage cars. I'd never have the bank balance for either but it's amazing how they reinforced my Fauntleroy image when casually left on my bed whilst I went on walkabout.

And walkabout, I did.

This was a key part of my time-killing strategy. Sometimes I'd just take a book down to Starbucks and read for an hour or so, nursing an Americano, pretending to be a visitor. Other times, I'd wander around the shop. I had no need for anything. It was just something more normal to do, rather than watching frail bodies struggling to repair themselves.

The shop near the main hospital entrance was about as far as I ventured. I was Tom Hanks in *The Terminal*. Pretty much free to roam any of the public spaces, just unable to leave. That's not strictly true. There was nothing to stop me from walking out and getting into a taxi. Certainly, no physical restraints. Not that it ever crossed my mind to leave. Where would I have gone anyway? Certainly not home. Karina would have removed my bollocks and pickled them in front of my eyes. I don't care what cheese it's served with, that's not a dish any man wants to try.

But my absolute belief was that even with all its apparent discombobulation, this was the best place for me. One patient in the opposite bay had taken some clothes to the bathroom, got changed, walked out of the building, and got a taxi home. He later phoned to say he was discharging himself. He'd even still had a cannula in each arm.

Three days later he was re-admitted and could barely breathe never mind walk. Sometimes you just have to take your medicine and shut up.

Another reason I was keen to spend time off the ward was down to my fellow patients. I'd seen a lot of faces in a variety of pre and post-operative states and care. All of which was a constant reminder of what could be coming my way.

Pretty much everyone in my bay and the one opposite was in for open-heart surgery. The specifics beyond that varied patient to patient, but everyone could look forward to the buzz saw separating their breastbone and their ribs being opened like the doors on a drinks cabinet.

The day before an operation, a familiar routine unfolded. There was the final visit from the surgeon; the chat about the goals and expectations of the surgery; the risks were discussed, and the consent forms were signed. The talky phase was followed by a benign activity which always gave me a chill.

A nurse would pull the curtains around the patient followed by the sound of an electric razor. Nobody brought it up, but everyone knew what was going on. The guy was being shaved from his neckline to his ankles, in readiness for the surgeon's knife. To me, there were parallels to shaving a convict's head to get better connectivity, prior to going to the Chair. But possibly, I was reading too much into it.

That said, this often took place during visiting hours so even visitors only a few feet away, knew what was going on, behind the thinnest of curtains. An old guy was getting a Brazilian from a young nurse. Not an image everyone is comfortable with.

Then the curtains are pulled back. There'd be a bit more chat; hugs, kisses, and wishes of good luck, promises to visit as soon as allowed and then they'd go. The guy is left on his bed, waiting for the clock to tick down. Alone.

I was always amazed at how calm and resigned they appeared, given what they were about to go through. I couldn't imagine I'd feel like that. After all, we'd all been witness to the same sights and sounds of very poorly and recovering patients on the ward. Previews of what was coming our way.

There's a subconscious impact when you see others go through something you'll shortly go through yourself. What's more, the impact is a double-edged sword. On one hand, your eyes are wide open to what to expect. The physicality of what awaited on the other side of the operation unfolded in front of me, day after day, so I had a point of reference. I knew what to expect, which is mostly a good thing. Generally, it's when there's a knowledge vacuum we tend to worry. We fill the vacuum with dark thoughts, rather than actual knowledge, which is why 90% of what we worry about, never happens.

The not so positive is... it's all very well knowing what's coming but when what's coming is a whole world of hurt, it doesn't sit so well. We all knew that the world of hurt was the ol' *short term pain for long term gain* thing. The challenge was (to use sales speak) tricking yourself to see beyond the features and look to the advantages and benefits. My problem was, I was always shit at sales. That, and the fact that I was surrounded by an awful lot of short-term pain.

Patients who, pre-op, had been chatty, lay motionless or were propped in their chair, barely speaking. There were drains stitched into their chests; a urine bag hooked to the underside of the bed meant there was a catheter embedded in their urethra; pacing wires were stitched into their torsos, and chest wound dressings were often visible. God knows what the actual wound looked like.

After a few days patients were encouraged to start moving around. Almost all were provided with Zimmer frames and shuffled along with their drainage bags of deep red liquid hooked onto the side of the frames. Nurses and Physios encouraged them to lift their feet, to stand upright and look ahead, rather than slouching and looking at the floor. Everything was such a visible effort.

Sometimes wounds became infected, adding another dimension to the level of care required. Most also had vein-harvest wounds in one or both legs. I saw such patients propped up in their chairs, their legs hugely swollen with trapped liquid from below the knee, with the wounds often weeping for several days.

Then there were the episodes of pain or sudden fluctuations in heart rate – all of which is very common following heart surgery. Breathing difficulties required prolonged periods on $O^2$ or a nebuliser. There was occasionally the need to have a pacemaker fitted several days after an operation and rarer still, people became so ill, they had to go back into theatre for further emergency surgery. Perhaps a new valve had failed, or a graft had become, I don't know, ungrafted. It was difficult to say as we often didn't see these patients again. In all probability, they would have been fine. A hospital ward doesn't operate like a hotel. You don't return to the same bed location you were in a week prior. But us remaining patients would never know, creating that knowledge vacuum which we all duly filled with our worst fears.

Post-operative patients were also tasked with lung exercises, using a plastic gadget of three short tubes each with a ball inside, attached to a long air tube. The patient sucked through the long tube to try and raise the three balls. It looked like a cross between an Andean Windpipe and a Bong. And judging by the difficulty and pain experienced by patients attempting the exercise, it was as challenging as it would've been to play.

Don't get me wrong, I also saw the progress of patient recovery, which in some cases was remarkable. Often, the shufflers became freestyle walkers within a matter of days. There were still drains and pacers attached, but they were carrying them themselves; they became chatty again and generally began re-engaging with the world. I was staggered at how quickly some of these, clearly, much older guys, were making progress. Seeing them, genuinely gave me hope and helped to offset images of the earlier stages of recovery.

One guy particularly enjoyed his recovery phase. He ordered a Chinese banquet for one, three nights running and this started only five days after his bypass. I don't know what impressed me more: that he had the gall and sense of independence to stand up to the institution to sort out this kind of treat for himself, or that the delivery guy managed to find the correct bed to deliver to. We're always getting our neighbours' takeaway drivers knocking on our door. If they can't find the correct house, how could Uber Eats find a bed? I salute both patient and driver.

# 11

## Couldn't Run A Bath

*"The best advice I've ever received is,*
*'No one else knows what they're doing either.' "*
**Ricky Gervais**

The rhythm and routine continued day after day. Doctors did their rounds. Some started at my end of the ward, some at the other, so I was either all done straight after breakfast or was tied to my bed until late morning. Waiting for the chance to move onto the next square of the game.

The rounds usually comprised a pair of Doctors, the Ward Sister and one of the nurses covering our bay. Sometimes very junior Doctors were present too. Students probably. Eager beavers, yet untainted by the impact of years of double shifts and the social life of a mole. The combinations of Doctors varied quite a bit and often, a completely new face would appear, which always made my heart sink.

I'm sure they were very competent Doctors, but a new face meant they had no retained idea of my back story - or in their terminology, my history; my symptoms - or how I had presented in medispeak; or where my story was going. New Face would flick through my notes and in quite matter of fact, but semi-authoritarian tones say things like, 'So, you were admitted following a heart attack, and it looks like you're being scheduled for a CABG – how are you today? Still having chest pain?'

'No, I have no chest pain. I've never had any chest pain, at any point. And I didn't have a heart attack. I was treated for a possible mild heart attack but -'

'Your notes say you had a heart attack.'

'Do they? Have you got the results of my Angiogram?'

'Angiogram? Errr...' furiously flicking through pages. 'No, I don't seem to be able to locate those. What did that show?'

'That came back as no heart attack but they found the blockage, hence the bypass, although apparently the MDT are discussing whether stenting is still an option.'

'*Are* they? Well, you have got a lot going on Mr Perry. So... no chest pain, breathing OK, O$^2$ sats are fine...'

At this point, the Ward Sister usually intervened and explained they were hoping for clarification of which route would be taken within the next few days and I was still going through the pre-op tests. New Face would then express his happiness with everything, bid his farewells and move on to the next patient, no doubt to dispense further pearls of wisdom.

These sorts of interactions were incredibly frustrating. I kept it bottled but it was there. I wanted to see progress but was delivered procrastination. Or so it felt.

Mostly though, there were combinations of Doctors who did know my (hi)story but still brought no news on what route would be taken. Again, fuel for the fire of frustration. The occasional test was initiated which I suppose felt like some progress was being made, even if the progress was glacial. But the overriding sensation was one of frustration.

The difficulty with having different combinations of Doctors was that the information each Doctor provided, varied so greatly. In my case, the variable information was usually down to their estimations on how long particular procedures would remain effective and therefore beneficial to me. I just wanted to know, how long a solution would last before another solution would be needed.

Inconsistent information? Guess what feeling that generates? Yup. Clever you. The compound effect of the F-word can be exponential. Especially when you throw in a measure of fear. Not the *swimming with sharks* kind of fear. But knowing your future life experiences are dependent on decisions made in the here and now, introduces a level of fear. You don't want to get them wrong by making decisions based on duff information. Although in fairness, *all* our future life experiences are largely dependent on everyday decisions we make in the here and now. We just tend not to overthink those everyday decisions.

I had a lot of time on my hands which meant a lot of Google time. I was determined to find out as much as I could about my condition, or various conditions; what the various clinical options were; their relative pros and cons; their success rates and the duration of their effectiveness. The last two aspects were of particular interest. I wanted black and white facts and numbers, so I knew I was comparing apples with apples and not apples with apple pie.

Just how long does a LAD bypass last? How long will a valve repair last? When could I expect to have further work done if I did have the repair? If I didn't have the repair, would it get worse and result in a complete valve replacement at some point? How long would a stent last? I'd seen that some could last for decades. Would further ablation work really improve my AF? The procedure on 1st March had done the complete opposite.

Medics don't provide guarantees. They don't deal in absolutes. Some Doctors would say 10-15 yrs for a bypass, others 20 to a lifetime. Some would say 10 years for a valve repair, others would say 20 to yet another lifetime. Confidence was even vaguer on the ablation. Maybe there would be no improvement at all, but everyone stressed they'd certainly want to avoid causing any unnecessary damage.

No shit Sherlock. I think the same thing when I'm parking my car, but the consequences are a little different.

I wanted specifics and guarantees so I could carry out the arithmetic. It sounds so obvious now, but to some extent, I was the architect of my own frustration. The variation is largely down to the patient, not the procedure.

I was also chasing the outcome from the MDT meeting. Daily. And that wasn't forthcoming either. Apparently, they'd met several times and each time my case had come up, more tests and information had been requested. Frustrations were rising and *the decision* had become almost the sole topic of conversation I had with anyone on the end of a text/WhatsApp/Messenger/email/phone call/visit.

Wednesday 1ˢᵗ May arrived. A pinch and a punch for the first of the month. Which, by coincidence, was what someone was going to get unless I got a decision on the solution pretty sharpish. I'd been in the second hospital for exactly one week, having been told after my Angiogram that an urgent bypass would be booked in for the following week. Still no decision. And on top of that, a Bank Holiday weekend was approaching. That would be my third consecutive Bank Holiday in hospital, and I was all too aware what happened in hospitals over Bank Holidays. The thin end of the *shit-all* wedge.

So, it was with eagerness I awaited a visit from a Doctor that day, as I'd heard the MDT had met again. He arrived with the usual entourage. There was the briefest of small talk, and then he got down to business.

'You'll be glad to know the MDT has come to a consensus on the way forward.'

'Excellent – what's the decision?'

'They've decided either way is a viable solution, so they're happy for you to decide.'

A pause hung in the air, waiting to be filled.

I was expecting to be told the experts were putting my money on either red or black. Not to be asked to make the gamble myself. All this time had passed, and they still couldn't, or now it appears, *wouldn't* decide.

I'd been brought up in quite a polite household, where manners had been valued and there was probably still some residual deference to authority figures. I think I've always managed to push that boundary whenever I've felt it needed to be pushed, but as a rule of thumb, I do so whilst still respecting the authority element. In short, ranting at coppers, or in this case Doctors, wasn't my default factory setting.

The pause was filled.

'I'm sorry, but that's just bollocks,' I spat.

The Sister quickly pulled the curtain around the bed, which cleverly not only made us invisible to other patients but also meant they couldn't hear us. Apparently.

I continued with my feedback.

'There's a reason why you lot went to school that liiiiiiiiiii-ttle bit longer than me... and that's to make decisions about what's best for the patient. How am I supposed to know what's best for me?' To amplify my point, I made the same gesture with my thumb and forefinger, that the Angiogram Consultant had made, when telling me a stent was not an option.

The conversation which followed was less conversation and more me venting that, by then, I'd been in hospitals for two weeks and no one was *owning* my case. I like to use that word when I feel people have turned their back on their duty and responsibilities. It suggests they're not just crap in their role, but that they've actively chosen to *avoid* the responsibility that comes with the role. One is a skills shortage, the other is attitudinal. I find it tends to smart more and provoke more of a response.

And it did, as he then offered his opinion - and he stressed it was only his opinion - which was he thought surgery would be the best option for someone of my age and general health, with my conditions.

Excellent – now we were getting somewhere. I shared that I was leaning towards that too but wanted some clarity on the valve repair as I'd had so many different estimates on how long it could last. His opinion was the repair should be good for life - which really just means a very long time and more than 5 to 10 years - but he'd get a second opinion.

I was happy with that and had the grace to apologise for having told him he was talking bollocks. He understood my frustrations and agreed that two weeks was a long time to be wandering around hospitals so 'bollocks' was a fair summation. I felt we parted as equals. No doubt he felt we parted as Doctor and shithead.

The following day, a Surgeon's second opinion confirmed that a valve repair of my nature should be good for decades and on 3$^{rd}$ May I advised the same Doctor my decision was for surgery. That was it – job done. No shortcuts or comfy chairs. No dodging hard time in favour of tidying my bedroom. A load lifted off my shoulders immediately. Strange how knowing once and for all that you're going to be cut open, your heart and lungs stopped, and you'll be put on a bypass machine, can bring so much serenity.

Nurse - sternum saw, please.

Having gone through the hoops of the previous two weeks, there was less anticipation of the Doctor's rounds the following day. I was in no rush to see them. The decision had been made. I could hazard a guess they wouldn't know the date yet, but it wouldn't be long. The mood was chipper in my neck of the woods.

Funny how when you're not desperate for attention, it comes quite quickly. The ward rounds arrived at my bed at 9:15. I hadn't seen this particular Doctor before and he had a couple of students with him, along with the usual Sister and nurse.

Pleasantries were exchanged, and he asked how I was. Naturally, I said how much better I felt now the decision had finally been made.

'What decision is that?'

'That I've decided on surgery rather than stenting.'

'Errr, there's no record of that here. Who made that decision?'

'I did. Why?'

'It's not really your decision to make and besides (looking at my notes), I think that's a little premature. We still need to discuss if surgery is the best option for you and what, if anything, should be done about the valve.'

And just like that, the atom was split. For the second time in 48 hours, the Sister reverted to rapid response tactics and drew the curtains around my bed, almost just by swiping her hand, it was that quick. Phew. Thank goodness other patients didn't hear what followed.

This guy knew nothing about my case. He hadn't seen my Angiogram report, my ultrasound scans, hadn't gone through the thread of discussions from the MDT. He was clearly *not* in possession of any relevant facts about me, whatsoever and therefore his opinion carried absolutely no weight with me at all. He should really move on to the next patient... I politely explained to him, using no bad language at all. (This is a lie.) The Sister did intervene at one point to assure the guy that Mr Perry had discussed the options at length with various Doctors and confirmed a decision had in fact, been made.

I saw my moment.

'Yes, it has! The decision I've made is that my case is being handled by Fuckwads.'

That's all I remember with any clarity. Apparently, I told the assembled medics they couldn't run a bath never mind a ward. It was the patient in the next bed who afterwards, told me I'd said this. I've been known to deploy the 'couldn't run a bath' phrase on occasion, so I can believe I said it, even if I can't recall it.

I continued to share my dissatisfaction with the shoddy progress made over the previous 2 ½ weeks. To be honest, the red mist was all about, and I can't recall the specific insults, but I left nothing in the pram. It was probably a bit pathetic really, but I felt abandoned. That I'd had no champion and was just adrift in their system. And not just adrift but drifting at their pace rather than the pace I'd been led to believe was required for my condition. A week and a half earlier I'd been told I needed treatment urgently, but by that stage, it was all beginning to sound a bit like:

'Hey let's do something!'

'Yeah... let's!'

'Ok... what?'

'Let's leave it to someone else to decide...'

'Excellent decision – that's what I would have done...'

The students were wide-eyed but doing everything they could to avoid eye contact with me. No doubt they were curious to see how their mentor would deal with this shithead of a patient. Trying to drag myself back to a point whereby progress of some sort could be made, I pointed out I'd been told that a Surgeon – a Mr D, was going to visit me the day before, to talk through what the surgery would entail. (See - we were that far down the road!) He obviously hadn't visited me so, I suggested we had that conversation later that day.

I was told Mr D now wouldn't be in until Tuesday 7th May, what with Monday being another Bank Holiday, which I knew, meant *nothing* would happen on my case. By then it was Saturday, 4th May. Star Wars day. Upon hearing that the surgeon had parked me on the other side of his Bank Holiday, my inner Jedi Warrior was roused, and major carnage was about to be unleashed. The Imperial NHS forces sensed this too and knew the invisibility curtains wouldn't be enough to contain the damage. The Doc quickly followed up by offering to phone Mr D, to see if he'd come in that weekend. Just to see me. Only me.

A bold attempt at diffusing the situation. But I knew better. I recognised an orderly retreat when I saw one. Why would a Consultant come in just to see me? He wasn't even on call and almost certainly had other plans for his Bank Holiday weekend. Family stuff. Or possibly golf. Definitely golf. Back in St Andrews again, with all the other Consultants. The bastard.

Having waited so long for a decision to be made and the serenity that follows in the aftermath of making such a massive decision, normal service had been resumed. Today's fuckening. The peace had been shattered. The patient, emotionally battered and faith in the NHS system, tattered. I asked to be left alone, which none of them could comply with quick enough, except the Ward Sister who mouthed a silent, 'Sorry'.

Being an atheist, I don't use the word *miracle* lightly. But at 10:15am, one happened. The Doc turned up with the Ward Sister and the talented Mr D. The main man. Le Grande Fromage. Apparently one of the best heart surgeons in the country. Although, I've heard it said, if you ask a heart surgeon for the names of the top three heart surgeons in the country, after pondering for a couple of minutes, they'll tell you they're struggling to think of the other two.

Mr D had something about him though. Not especially tall but blessed with a youthful face that belied his years. He had a natural air of authority. Here was someone who was too busy and frankly, too damn talented to skirt around the edges of an issue. He immediately offered an apology for all the confusion and said the hospital hadn't handled my situation very well. If nothing else, he'd been well briefed.

He went on to provide some detail and maintained that either solution could work – stenting or surgery. He reiterated my Mitral Valve wasn't at a stage where they'd ordinarily consider replacing it or even repairing it, noting though that it may continue to deteriorate, or it may not.

He was very confident the valve repair could last *a very long time*. I was fixated on the duration of the solution by this stage. I was looking for reassurance I wouldn't be back in 5-10 years.

Further ablation – trying to correct the erroneous electrical signals causing the AF - had been mentioned in some early conversations but all the recent focus had been on the solution for the narrowed artery and whether a valve repair should be carried out.

Mr D put a different spin on it. He saw the potential for further ablation as a significant factor in the final decision and stressed its importance. He'd already requested information from Gordon, regarding the previous procedure, wanting to know if there were any more options to remove or reduce the AF. If a solution for the AF was viable, this would be a strong case for surgery. If there was little point in further ablation, surgery may not be the best way forward. In his eyes, stopping the AF could help the performance of the Mitral Valve.

I discovered shortly after this conversation, the reason why my case had landed on his desk was that he was one of the few surgeons who specialised in all three procedures: CABG, valve work and ablation.

For the first time in this whole 2 ½ week journey, I felt like I was getting somewhere. I was being presented with rational, clear information based on joined-up thinking and it felt good. But then a thought came to mind.

'But if this is what you're thinking today, on Saturday, then the conversations I had on Wednesday and since then, have all been - ' and simultaneously we both said, 'premature.' I made the point that the time spent deliberating had been a complete waste of time, energy, and anxiety, as I'd had inaccurate information. He completely agreed and apologised again, on behalf of the hospital.

Mr D was now owning this case and I was grateful for that. Despite me having psychologically readied myself for open-heart surgery and in my lay way, felt it was the better longer-term solution, he was suggesting we may end up with a far less invasive intervention. He was at pains to point out his mind was far from decided and said many times, that there are so many grey areas. He would have the information he required later that day; would review it over the weekend and meet with me again on Tuesday.

He then turned to the Sister and requested that my pre-operative tests be fast-tracked for before the Tuesday meeting, so he had all the results to consider. Once again, it felt like things were on the move and although I was still in the dark as to what the outcome would be, my case was at least in the spotlight of someone who was going to see it through to its conclusion.

As the conversation was wrapping up so amicably, I thought it only fair to apologise to the other Doc who had been on the receiving end of my verbal Dogs of War. (This was becoming a habit.) He may well have known very little about the specifics of my case, but he knew no decision had been made, so had been totally correct in that respect. In turn, he apologised once again, for the confusion the hospital had caused.

Once they'd both left, the Sister said she'd arrange the tests for as soon as possible and told me she thought I'd spoken very eloquently and completely understood my frustration, which was nice of her. I could only assume she wasn't referring to the conversation which had taken place about an hour before. Although she did say she loved my *couldn't run a bath* line and would be stealing it for herself. That was nice too.

# 12

## Demob Happy

*"Experience is the hardest kind of teacher.*
*It gives you the test first and the lesson afterwards."*
**Oscar Wilde**

The following day, I'd barely finished breakfast when a Porter arrived with the by then, all too familiar blue wheelchair. A nurse informed me I was being taken for a vein scan, so if they did have to harvest (I love that word in this context) a vein, they could be confident it'd be up to standard. It was only an ultrasound scan, so no biggie.

So soon after breakfast, I was still in my pyjama bottoms and was going to get dressed but was told I was fine as I was. I was the first to be scanned that day and the nurse didn't want me to cause any delay. Fair enough.

I'm eventually wheeled into a dimly lit consultation room with a bed, the ultrasound machine, and an operator. I perched myself on the edge of the bed. The operator was a young woman in her mid-20s wearing scrubs and even in the poor lighting, I could see she had an impressive jungle of tattoos around her right arm. Excuse me for noticing but she wasn't unattractive and had a scent about her that wasn't entirely unpleasant. There was a bit of chit chat... and was that a slight Irish lilt?

Ok. She was really quite attractive and smelt lovely. Even her tats had something about them. (Yes, that is the vowel I meant to use.) But it was inappropriate to think that way; after all, we were both professionals and had a job to do. Even if mine was just to lay there and not be a pest. She asked if I had any tattoos on my legs. I thought we were still in the chit-chat phase so said I hadn't got around to my legs yet. Or indeed anywhere. It got a smile but it appeared the question was clinically based as obviously, my artwork may become distorted should a vein be removed.

She was sitting on a stool in front of the scanning unit entering some patient info and eventually swivelled round to face me, indicating she was ready to start. I'd seen plenty of guys on the ward either with bandages on the lower legs or seen the wounds themselves, so swung my legs up onto the bed and pulled my pyjamas up past my knees.

'Ah... no. I'm going to need you to stand on this small step and for you to lower your pyjamas,' she said, almost apologetically.

'I'm sorry, what?' was my reflex reply. There must've been some confusion. Her request was casting doubt on my understanding of where the vein would be taken from. She clearly read my confusion.

'I'm sorry but I need to scan your whole leg.'

My whole leg? I'd thought they were checking in case they'd need a vein for a bypass... for me... not for everyone on the ward.

'They'd just take it from below the knee, wouldn't they?' There was more than a touch of pleading to my tone.

'They'll take it from above the knee, but we need to be confident the whole leg vein is OK.' There was a slight beat. 'I'm really sorry.'

The cold, unavoidable reality of what was about to happen, was sinking in. I was going to have to drop my jimmies, in front of this, quite attractive young woman sitting in front of me, whilst I stood on a footstool, fully exposed.

It crossed my mind to try and fill the uncomfortableness with something witty like, 'Wouldn't it be fairer if we were both naked?' but then thought that might involve statements, lots of paperwork, and having to sign a register, so parked that one.

But picture this; I'm standing on a ten-inch stool in front of this young woman (did I mention she was quite attractive?) who has a heavily gelled ultrasound probe and is slowly and methodically working along the full length of my leg from deep within my groin to my ankle. Now to her credit, she stayed in role and wasn't distracted in any way, by what must have been, tantalisingly (my word, not hers) close to her face. She was capturing her measurements and repeated some areas at different angles, just as she had been trained to do. Meanwhile, I was cultivating a full-body, cold, clammy sweat and appeared to have left my dignity on the other side of the door. Perhaps I'd just mislaid it? I didn't recall handing it over or being mugged.

It was excruciating – mentally, not physically. Although there were some notable physical responses beyond prolific sweating, one of which, I felt didn't present me in the kindest of lights. Another one was my throat, which had begun to dry up. I wanted to swallow but there was nothing to swallow. In the absence of being able to swallow, I began to feel the need to cough. But knew if I did, there would be a high chance the reverb would cause a flick of the jonk right against this woman's face. In the space of a nanosecond, she'd suffer PTSD and I'd be embroiled in an assault charge.

If I'd thought my banter might have generated some paperwork, imagine what a jonk-to-face incident would do. Christ my veins had better be bloody good. Finally... she finished, and it was all over. I was about to be reunited with my dignity and couldn't reach down for my jimmies quick enough.

That's when she said, 'Now the right leg,' which sent me into a spasm of coughing causing my tackle to bounce into some sort of freestyle, hip-hop routine.

In light of this development, it was so thoughtful of her to ask if I needed any water; the offer of which I gratefully accepted. She stepped over to the water butt, filled a paper cup and passed it to me. It would have been kind of weird to temporarily pull my jimmies back up, over the cloggy gel still coating my left leg, just to drink some water and then have to pull them down again for the right leg to be scanned.

But possibly not as weird as staying putt on the stool, trousers down, tackle out, tipping water down my throat so fast it was running down my chest, over my groin and onto my legs, whilst a young woman sat in front of me, patiently waiting, in a dimly lit room. Which of course, is exactly what happened.

I appreciate some people pay good money for this sort of experience but whatever route the medical team ultimately decided on, I decided, the worst must surely be over. I also appreciate women undergo all manner of intimate examinations every few years, often carried out by male Doctors. The difference is, they may have a few years to psychologically prepare themselves. Whereas I'll be needing a few years to psychologically get over it.

True to his word, Mr D arrived at 9:20am on Tuesday 7th May, along with Gordon, who explained that he was the Sparky and Mr D was the Plumber. Two for the price of one. A double act – excellent. I made a mental note to check their reviews on TrustATrader.com. They got straight to the point.

They shared the opinion that the blockage was the main issue, but both were also optimistic my AF could be addressed with further ablation work. This meant they favoured surgery. So, whilst the bypass graft was non-negotiable, it would have been remiss not to repair the valve, whilst in there. What's more, they were very much of the opinion that all these treatments combined - which they referred to as whole heart 'remodelling' - would all benefit each other. Once the information had been imparted, Mr D said his farewells and shot off to another plumbing job leaving Gordon and me to talk some more.

'Mr D's not one for small talk, but if it were me or anyone in my family needing the operation, I'd want him to do it. And unless it was an absolute emergency, I'd be prepared to wait for him to become available.'

High praise indeed, from The Police frontman. Once again, I began to feel grateful to be in such competent hands, with Specialists who were owning my situation and offering a solution to allow me to get on with my life. It wasn't just the previous 2-3 weeks. It felt like this *thing* had been hanging over me for the last 2-3 years since the AF had first been diagnosed. Finally, it looked like there was a way out.

The relief was immense. My shoulders were dropping.

Gordon also stressed the aim of the combined surgical treatments was to allow me the active life I desperately wanted – to be able to have a great quality of life – not to just *get by*.

*Yes! Yes! Yes! This was exactly what I wanted! Let's go – get me in there now!*

That's when he broke the news that, as I'd already been in hospital(s) for the best part of three weeks and had been completely stable, I couldn't be classed as a medical emergency anymore. It'd probably be another two-to-three weeks at least, before my operation date.

'But what about the ticking time bomb?'

It was all relative apparently. Yes, this repair needed carrying out very soon but theatres needed to be prioritised for transplants and other screaming emergencies.

This was a blow after the high of getting the green light on surgery. Maybe not so much a blow as an amber light. We'd be proceeding, just not at lightning pace. It seemed there was no continuous, straight upwards path of progress in matters of health. But then, I shouldn't have been surprised. Since when has *life* been one continuous, straight upward path of progress? Maybe it's the bumps in the road and turbulence on the flight that make the arrival more appreciated.

In the meantime, Gordon pondered whether I really wanted to be stuck in hospital for a further 2-3 weeks, waiting for an operation? Did he really need to ask that question? I couldn't wait to get out! They clearly needed the bed and considered I was in no immediate danger, so it was agreed I was to be put on short-term release and discharged.

There were a few conditions attached to this short-term release. Although I'd been completely stable, I'd been doing virtually nothing but walking around the whole time, so was told to try and keep it that way at home. This was not to be seen as an opportunity to cut the hedges, go for long bike rides or walk in the hills. The message was, take it easy and all would be fine. It appeared Karina and I were finally going to make a start on *Game of Thrones*.

Karina was keen to get me home too. Visiting hospital for most of the day, every day was beginning to take its toll, which I could completely understand. Apart from all the practical stuff such as meal management and keeping on top of the boys' revision, it was tough emotionally. Allocating most of your day to being out and thinking constantly about someone else, doesn't leave much time to get other things done or space in your own head for downtime.

I would have walked out there and then but had to wait for the Pharmacist to visit with a new set of meds. This is easier to arrange than to experience. I was fully packed up and ready to go from 10am and the nurses were keen to give the bed to someone more deserving than me. That said, they were also very grateful for the time I'd been in there as I'd been a *self-manager*. I'd not lost control of my bodily functions; required impromptu bedsheet changes; wandered to someone else's bed and tried to get in with them or steal their clothes. I'd not tried to discharge myself whilst connected to drips; fallen over going to or from the bathroom; locked myself in the toilet whilst shouting bingo numbers, sworn at other patients, their visitors, my own visitors or staff. That last one is obviously a bit of a porky, but it was a two-way street.

Neither had I thrown my food, ordered it from a Chinese Takeaway, or not eaten my food. I'd avoided MRSA, bedsores and hadn't exposed myself to patients, visitors or staff. (The leg vein scanner, aside.) Ultimately, I'd avoided becoming ill or dying.

The Sister on duty told me they'd miss me.

Awwww... I'd sort of got to know them too and would miss them a bit, as well.

She clarified what she meant. Because I'd needed no help and had generated no extra work, for two whole weeks, life had been, by comparison, a bit easier. It'd meant there'd been more time for the other five patients in the bay. The nurses' workload was about to go up by 20%, back to six, fully demanding patients. So, not quite the sentimental gesture I'd originally thought but I was glad to have been of incremental benefit to the other patients.

By 4:30 pm, (a record-breaking 6½ hrs later) the Pharmacist had been, I had my meds and Karina and I were getting outta Dodge.

One of the last things I had to do was complete a *Patient Satisfaction Survey*. It was only a short questionnaire of about five or six questions and was more ward focussed than on clinical outcomes. Answers had to be given on a five-point scale from a very sad emoji face up to a very smiley emoji face.

I'd imagine every ward issued these cards when patients were discharged. No doubt an idea masterminded by some marketing consultant who wouldn't dream of using the NHS out of choice.

There'd be a league table of wards somewhere, although it may have operated more along the lines of TripAdvisor. Remarkably, the final question asked, 'How likely are you to recommend this ward to family and friends?'

This is worth a moment or two of reflection. How likely was I to recommend this cardio-thoracic ward, to my family and friends?

Well...let me think. Not particularly that much if you'd just been looking for an Airbnb with good transport links, or perhaps if you'd been unlucky enough to have a brain or spinal injury. *But...* if you'd happened to have an issue of the cardio or indeed, thoracic nature, then yes, I'd say that my ward was indeed worthy of a very smiley face. On that basis, I would highly recommend it to family and friends. But as a general rule of thumb, if you can keep a shit load of distance between it and yourself, almost anywhere else, would be preferable.

And that's said with the utmost respect and gratitude for those who cared for me there.

I'd been in hospitals for three weeks and as weird as it sounds, I did feel a little disorientated on the journey home. Karina noticed I was a bit quiet and asked about it. I think I may have been suffering from early-stage, onset institutionalisation. It was strange to drive past places I recognised and to have the freedom of being outside the hospital.

Our home felt very familiar though. It was lovely to see the boys again under normal circumstances, in normal surroundings, having normal conversations. After dinner, I watched some football with them but we chatted over it, most of the time. It was just lovely to be back at home and going to sleep in our own bed was just bliss.

One of the things I missed whilst in hospital was a lie-in. Being woken every day, so perfectly clean bedsheets could be replaced, meant the luxury of the lie-in had never been an option for the last three weeks. Not that I would've got much of one on weekdays anyway, but I'd missed three weekends and three bank holidays. That's nine potential days for a few extra hours in bed. I bet the rest of the country had taken advantage.

So, when the sun rose on 8th May, for the first time in three weeks, I didn't have to get up with it and I slept through to gone nine. And it was bloody brilliant. I felt great.

Karina had been downstairs sorting the boys' breakfasts. They'd both gone off to school and college and she came upstairs sometime around 9:30am with a mug of tea for each of us. We talked about the madness of the last three weeks and what we were going to do that day. Given the restrictions imposed, we were moving towards a gentle walk in our local park, where we'd grab a coffee.

Now that the decision on surgery had been made and I was out of hospital, I felt light and liberated. My medical team had a thorough plan on how to fix me for the long term. I was free of the burden of not knowing what was going to happen. The sun was shining and I felt incredibly optimistic. It was going to be a great first full day back in relative normality.

That was the last thing I remember. After the huge wins of my medical team formulating a roadmap for my recovery, the decision for surgery, and going home to wait for it, suddenly I lost. Big time.

The biggest loss of all.

# 13

## Karina: Not On My Watch

*"Enjoy yourself. It's later than you think."*
**Herb Magidson**

Finally, the luxury of a slow morning and a lie-in. We were chatting about a park walk and visiting the café for our usual take-out coffees. A total break from the hospital routine – happy days! But first, another cup of tea was needed, no need to rush after all, or so I thought.

I briefly glanced away from Karl... and then looked back. In those few seconds, *it* happened. Or rather *something* had already started. Karl was looking up at the ceiling, beyond me, his face contorted. I totally expected him to break away from this at any second, and for us to carry on with our chat about morning plans.

That didn't happen. I couldn't really process or understand what I was seeing. It wasn't making any sense. Karl wasn't moving or responding, his eyes were open but not blinking, as if in a trance. It took a few more seconds, but then the horror of the realisation that something was very seriously wrong, hit me.

I grabbed his phone from his bedside cabinet. So lucky it was there and charged; not something we were always good at. I hit the emergency button and prayed it would connect. It did and I was put through to the ambulance service. I can't recall how the call handler introduced herself but let's call her Angela. She asked questions and I rattled through what I was seeing, in a very shouty, frantic, desperate manner. She had her work cut out.

She told me to calm down; that she was trying to help me but couldn't unless I got a grip. It wasn't put quite that way, but I got the message. It cut through my chaos and I regained some composure. Having a similar address not too far away from us where post, pizzas, curries and the like have previously been lost to, I knew I had to convey our address very clearly. They weren't having this ambulance as well.

Having done so, Angela was now on a fact-finding mission. I explained the unfolding scene. Karl was now gasping for breath, yet still unconscious and motionless. I had no idea what was happening. She asked where he was – on the bed, I said – she told me to remove the pillows so he was flat and to start CPR immediately.

'What?!' I shouted in disbelief. I had absolutely no idea what to do, or how to do it. Calmly and gently, Angela told me she'd talk me through it. And she did. Her air of authority was comforting. I followed her instructions to the letter; interlocking my hands, one on top of the other, I placed them in the middle of Karl's chest, then started the compressions, hard and fast.

'Do *not* stop,' she said.

There was no catchy *Stayin' Alive* Bee Gees tune to keep me company. Instead, I followed Angela's beat, as she called the count down the phone:

1-2, 1-2, 1-2...

About two compressions a second. She kept on repeating it, over and over again:

1-2, 1-2, 1-2...

Anyone who's done CPR will know how exhausting it is. I was using my shoulders and arms to push down as hard and deep as I could with all my weight. Apparently, this is a good technique. Who knew?! Karl being on a bed however was not so good! It didn't register at the time, but CPR on a mattress, absorbing some of the compression, wasn't the ideal place for efficiency. Probably best that I was oblivious to this. I had no idea as to whether any of this was working or not.

1-2, 1-2, 1-2... on and on and on.

After a short time, I told Angela I didn't think it was making a difference. She insisted that it was and that I just had to keep going.

1-2, 1-2, 1-2...

During all of this, the phone which I'd pinned between my ear and shoulder, leaving my hands free for the compressions, was starting to slip. That triggered another panic. Placing it on the bed and switching it to loudspeaker, I was certain I'd knock the call off. Remarkably my clumsy gene didn't kick in and I carried on with the 1-2s.

Angela wanted to know if anyone was in the house with me. I told her I was on my own. Our fabulous boys had left for school and college earlier that morning. She asked if the front door was locked. I said it was closed, but not locked. Was that the same thing?

1-2, 1-2, 1-2...

She kept breaking off and seemed to repeatedly ask if the door was definitely unlocked. I didn't understand why she kept referring to it. Not much was making sense anymore... so much chat about the door. Although I did wonder how on earth the Paramedics would be getting in.

Karl's eyes had become fixed and the gasping had stopped. I was now shouting that all this *JUST WASN'T WORKING*. Then the news I was desperate for; the Paramedics were close and I'd hear the ambulance soon. Unbeknown to me, two ambulances were racing from different locations.

Angela, with all the calmness of the calmest of all calm people, told me that very soon when she shouted, 'Run' I'd have to stop the CPR, get downstairs and open the door for the Paramedics. The *door* penny dropped! And that filled me with dread. What would I find on my return?

I heard the sirens. They were becoming louder and louder, closer and closer. It was quite possibly the most glorious sound I'd ever heard. Angela warned me she was going to ask me to run at any second. I was exhausted and desperately needed them to arrive.

And then the call came:

R-U-N!!

I've felt nothing like it. The urgency of having to run. Losing balance, bumping into furniture, slipping down the stairs, flinging the door open... and there he was. The guy in green. The cavalry had well and truly arrived. Steve, (let's say) was now in charge and the relief was overwhelming. A professional had stepped in. Someone who knew what they were doing.

In seconds we were upstairs and lifted Karl, still unconscious, off the bed onto the floor. In a calm, confident and measured manner Steve began CPR.

My role then changed to *helper*. What could I do? What did he need? I got Steve the bits and bobs he asked for, from his bag. And then his companion, a second Paramedic arrived, let's call her Hannah. She was chatty and bubbly and asked what had happened. I gave an update and an outline of Karl's recent medical goings-on. Whilst they got on with looking after Karl, I managed to speak to my most wonderful Brother in law, Jus who lived locally and asked him to get hold of my gem of a sister, Sarah. Within what seemed like minutes she appeared. Teleportation must have been involved.

Meanwhile, in the background, chilling words came from the Paramedics, 'He's not breathing.' The paddles came out and were slapped onto Karl's chest. Seconds later a shock was administered.

He jolted but didn't respond.

I heard again, 'He's still not breathing.'

A second shock was delivered. Within a few seconds, Karl opened his eyes and started talking to Steve. He was answering questions and responding to requests.

Alert. Literally. Just like that.

Steve told him he'd had a cardiac arrest. This was the first time the term had been used. A few checks were run. The heart rhythm was confirmed as fine. The ECG was looking good. It was as if nothing had happened.

But then, that was always going to be the case, wasn't it? Bizarrely, this was the only outcome, despite my hysteria, that I expected. The driving force, as I was pounding away, desperately trying to keep Karl with us was, *I am NOT allowing this to happen - not on my watch.* I was not telling our boys, who'd been so happy to have their Dad home, the worst news possible. That had pushed me, driven me, and given me the strength to keep going.

Once I'd realised everything was 'OK' .... I suddenly transformed into the sociable host, bantering with Steve and Hannah. I wasn't far off asking if they wanted a cup of tea and a chocolate digestive! The small talk just poured out of me. It was madness. Complete and utter madness.

It had taken 11 minutes for the ambulance to arrive. With Angela's brilliance and a lot of luck, I'd been able to keep Karl's heart in a shockable rhythm for Steve and Hannah to work their magic. I had no medical training and last went on a First Aid course in the last millennium (although CPR definitely wasn't included!), so I wasn't the best-equipped candidate to perform it. However, from this tale,

I'd hope the signs of cardiac arrest are now more understood and I'd encourage everyone to learn CPR. You never know. It might not just be someone else's life you're saving; it might be your own, too.

# 14

## Why So Miserable?

*"You're in pretty good shape, for the shape you are in."*
**Dr Seuss**

Coldness. As if I was wet but only on my back. Then another sensation came into focus. There was something on my face. Something covering my nose and mouth. I instinctively brought my hands up to brush it off. In doing so, other hands took hold of my wrists and arms and moved them away from my face. Then a noise. It took a few seconds before I could make sense of it... someone was talking to me. The stimuli were coming in quite quickly but in layers. I opened my eyes and became aware of a couple of people dressed in green. I could see I was laying on my back; one person, a man, was kneeling next to me on my right and the other, a woman, nearer my feet. I was pretty sure I was in our bedroom, next to our bed, laying on the floor. What I wasn't so sure about was, why and was it all real?

I had a vague recollection of being in hospital recently but thought I'd been discharged. Which meant this must all be a dream. A really vivid dream. But the talking, the coldness on my back and the thing on my face which, by then, I'd realised was an oxygen mask, all felt very real. Very quickly my thoughts leapt track. Perhaps it was the memory of being in hospital that was the dream. As I was considering this alternative perspective on events, I'd concluded the people in green were paramedics. This all took place in a matter of seconds. I looked to my left and saw the under-bed drawer which confirmed I was laying on our hard wooden bedroom floor. That explained the coldness. I could also see Karina and her sister, Sarah, standing near the dressing table, both looking mystifyingly upset. Why was Sarah in our bedroom? And why did they both look so upset? There was also a third, male Paramedic stood near the bedroom door.

My state of confusion was becoming resolved. Except for why. Why was I on my back? Why were Paramedics here? Not just Paramedics – three of them. My mind hit the rewind button. Paramedics didn't feature so, why were they here now? I was together enough to guess something serious had happened to me. But what? My recent memory rewind confirmed I'd felt well; I'd had no pain, no dizziness, no breathlessness...

My question was answered without being asked.

'Karl... Karl... can you hear me? You've had a cardiac arrest.'

I looked at the Paramedic talking to me. It was the nearest one. I nodded as if to say, 'Oh yea?' I was asked if I understood, and I nodded again.

I was asked my name, which I gave. I was asked if I knew where I was. I replied, my bedroom. I was then asked, where that was. What was the address? I replied with the house number and road name, for which I was rewarded with the kind of praise and tones usually reserved for puppies, toddlers, and residents of care homes.

At that point, I accepted their explanation for the scenario in a manner that can only be described as emotionless and clinical. I thought I understood what having a cardiac arrest meant – that your heart had stopped – and it's not often a heart restarts all by itself. In fact, it's so *not often*, it's *never*. If they were saying that's what had happened, I took it at face value. But I was doing so with a sense of; *but I'm awake, talking and feeling completely OK*. My thinking was becoming clearer by the second and I certainly wasn't feeling any pain. So, although accepting of the situation, I was also confused. A cardiac arrest is a terrible thing to happen to someone, but I was feeling pretty good, considering. I would have expected to have felt mighty shit after a cardiac arrest. How I felt, didn't chime with what I was being told.

As if to underline this point, when one of the Paramedics asked if I could give Karina a thumbs up, I recall doing it with gusto, not just making a thumb gesture by my side. I rolled slightly her way, turned to look, raised my arm, and gave the thumb directly to her.

This generated further toddler-dodderer praise, which to be fair, did make me feel quite good, which was probably the Paramedic's intention all along. That and to see what my motor skills were like. But as all was looking so good, I was fully expecting to be helped to my feet, dusted down, and told to sit out the rest of the day in front of Netflix.

Instead, I was transferred from the flat of the floor to a medivac chair, which I took as medical folk being overly cautious. I was prepared to humour them. *Game of Thrones* wasn't going anywhere. I could start it later that day.

Only then, in a slightly seated position, did I suddenly become acutely aware of considerable pain in my chest. Painful to the point it was difficult to get a full lungful of air. Pain which, in the course of a second, terrified me. Having just convinced myself that a cardiac arrest wasn't so bad after all, I wasn't shy about sharing my sudden awareness of pain which wasn't so much *in* my chest, as, *all over* it. I was told I had my wife to thank for that.

I was quickly reassured it was unlikely the source of the pain would be my heart. What I was feeling were *compression pains* from Karina pounding my chest trying to keep my heart going.

'Chances are, you'll have a few broken ribs. But look at it this way, if you're feeling pain, it means she did a good job,' said one of the Paramedics, chirpily.

I was lucid enough to interpret the real message and was apologising to Karina, having put her through it all. I was saying how awful it must have been for her. 'Yes, it fucking was and so you should be', would've probably been the honest response, but she appeared almost dismissive of her role.

Although I'd only been conscious for a few minutes, as I say, I'd been comfortably in the *this isn't as bad as it seems,* camp. Once it began to sink in that Karina had been pumping my chest, to the extent of possibly breaking my ribs, my position shifted.

This shifting position was quite starkly accentuated by the Paramedic who'd been closest to me. 'You're doing amazingly well Karl. In 16 years of doing this job, I've never seen someone come back so strongly, so quickly, immediately after a cardiac arrest.'

At that point, although I accepted something serious had happened, I can't say I fully processed the significance of what he was saying. I suppose I was encouraged I was not only doing well but was also extremely statistically abnormal - in a positive way. That's natural right? If someone says you're the best example they've ever seen of something, then that's got to be good. It's a compliment. Who wouldn't feel a bit gee-ed up on hearing something like that?

On the other hand, I was aware there was another, deeper meaning to what he was saying but my antennae were only vaguely picking it up. At best, it was probably coming through as, *so usually people don't feel this good after a cardiac arrest.* Which, while true, I now understand is like looking at the situation through the wrong end of a telescope. I also accepted I wouldn't be kicking back in front of *Game of Thrones*, anytime soon.

Yet even as I was picking up on the potential gravity of my situation, there was a juxtaposition with what was going on around me. Karina was enthusiastically talking with the female Paramedic about everyday things and our everyday lives. It was all so surreal.

I was wheeled down the stairs, wrapped in my blanket and strapped into the chair. I felt physically very safe but once outside, very exposed to neighbourly and passing eyes. Ambulances are much bigger than they look in your rear-view mirror and even bigger still, close up and parked outside your own house with blue lights flashing. Karina and the female Paramedic were still busy in animated, upbeat chat by the time I was on the drive. It was at odds with how I was feeling, by then. The joy of *the big win* had been replaced with the knowledge I'd taken a giant leap backwards. It's fair to say, I was a bit down in the mouth, at which point Karina looked at me with a puzzled face saying, 'Stop looking so miserable. Cheer up – you're alive, aren't you?'

What was this new reality I'd found myself in?

I was wheeled into the ambulance and Karina joined me inside. I was strapped in, and we set off to our local hospital at speed, with blue lights flashing and sirens wailing. Which even then, all seemed a bit unnecessary and over the top to us.

Apparently, others thought differently and there was still some urgency, after all.

# 15

# Doc Swagger

*"Do or do not. There is no try."*
**Yoda**

Whilst in the ambulance, the Paramedic was looking at my ECG printout and observed that, apart from my AF, he couldn't see anything hugely out of the ordinary, which appeared odd from his perspective but massively reassuring from ours. Once in A&E, I was rushed into a curtained bay and a Doctor was immediately briefed on my status. They weren't sparing the horses.

'So, Mr Perry, you've had an exciting start to the day. Bystander CPR? Remarkable.' But then addressed Karina. 'You did exceptionally well,' to which she just nodded quietly.

He continued reading through the notes provided by the Paramedics and I was asked about chest pain or discomfort, dizziness, shortness of breath etc. I answered, 'No' to all excepting, of course, for the compression pains.

'You're in a privileged position Mr Perry – only the lucky ones get to feel those,' he replied. 'We'll just make sure you're stable here but then we'll be transferring you. We'll run some tests, but I'd say you're in pretty good shape having had a cardiac arrest less than 30 minutes ago.'

Karina picked up the ECG printout laying on my bed and asked, 'How can you be sure he'll be stable because there isn't much to go on, on this ECG.'

'I don't doubt for one second that you've had a cardiac arrest but you're right, there's absolutely nothing on here suggesting a major cardiac incident.' He paused, looked at Karina and asked, 'Do you have a medical background?'

Karina explained that she didn't and it was just something the Paramedic had said.

'Ah, I just thought with that comment and the successful CPR that you were one of us. Remarkable.' At which point we were interrupted as a portable X-ray machine was brought to my bed. I was only in A&E for about 90 mins before being wheeled back into an ambulance for onward transfer back to the hospital I'd just been in for two weeks.

I can't recall too much about the transfer except that Karina came with me and the blue lights and siren were switched on. Something I again, felt wasn't particularly necessary, in my extensive medical opinion. Having arrived at the hospital, there was a short wait in the corridor outside of the Cardiac Care Unit whilst a bed was arranged.

Whilst waiting, the Paramedic who'd been with us inside the ambulance (but different from any of those who'd been in our house) looked down at me and said, 'You have no idea what an incredibly lucky outcome you've had today.'

I just nodded gently, saying, 'Yeah,' in response. I wasn't feeling particularly chatty. I had a very faint understanding of what he was getting at, but not with any great sense of gravity.

I was fairly quickly allocated a bed although, strictly speaking, it was a bay as that kind of facility isn't set up like a typical ward. It was far more open plan with the emphasis on flexibility of space. In case you need to be hooked up to a shedload of machinage to keep you going, I'd imagine.

I was slid over from the ambulance bed to the hospital bed and put in a sitting position. The sides were put up, the bed height was raised, and I was told to move as little as possible and to definitely *not* get out of bed. I was left some empty Californian Carafes, should I feel the urge. The Nurses' Station was in the centre of the room from where they could see every patient in the facility, even those in some of the private rooms as each room had large windows. The place felt more *special* than your average ward.

The Sister introduced herself and explained what would be happening next in terms of tests. All the usual suspects, but at some point, I'd have an echocardiogram (ultrasound) of the heart, which is not to be confused with an electrocardiogram (ECG) which I'd also been hooked up to. An echocardiogram doesn't appear to have a TLA (three-letter abbreviation), presumably because the electrocardiogram got there first in claiming ECG. Which begs the question, why didn't they just call an echocardiogram a cardiac ultrasound and abbreviate that to CUS? Missed a trick there, med folk. Imagine the seconds that could be shaved off sentences both written and spoken over the course of a day.

The Sister also advised that the next 24hrs were crucial and re-inforced the notion of moving as little as possible. My options for doing anything but that were narrow and although the instruction - it definitely wasn't advice or even a request - made sense given what had happened, the reference to the next 24hours hadn't been made clear to us, so we asked. Apparently, I was at my most vulnerable to some follow up cardiac incident during this time.

I can see why they'd been a little vague. Being told there was a possibility of after-shocks following the main quake, doesn't do a whole lot of good in the anxiety-lowering stakes.

A little later, a confident young Glaswegian Doctor approached my bed, flanked by two nurses. When I say confident, I mean he spoke at a volume above an indoor voice but not quite an outdoor voice. More of a *getting your coat off the peg in the cloakroom and heading to the playground* voice. There was a swagger to him too. If it's possible to swagger in scrubs. He was very much in *watch-and-learn* mode. The Sage on his personal stage.

They all introduced themselves and explained that one of the nurses was a student. The Doc was there to put an ART line in my arm and produced what looked like a spare guitar string from the tray the nurse was holding.

'A what?'

He gently chided himself for using an abbreviation and explained it was short for an Arterial Line or an Arterial Catheter. It meant that a wire could be fed through an artery in my arm, which would allow them to take blood pressure readings, but from much closer to my heart and on a real-time basis. It wouldn't hurt, in fact, I wouldn't feel a thing, he told me with the air of someone who did this kind of thing on autopilot. In his sleep. Without using his hands. That's just how good he was.

The needle went into my right arm, but after a bit of wiggling, he established he wasn't in an artery, requiring him to remove it, apply a ball of cotton wool and a plaster and try again. Again – he didn't strike oil. Another ball of cotton wool and a plaster were applied.

Let's try the left arm. In we go. No, we don't. Nurse... cotton wool. Plaster. Three shots and none on target.

Doc Swagger was becoming visibly frustrated and adopted the medic's classical defensive position in this type of situation, by shifting the blame onto the patient with the question, 'Ar ya usually this stingy when it comes ta sharin' yer arteries and veins?'

Naturally, I said no, but not in a way to antagonise him. He still needed to get a bloody needle into my arm. To be fair, he wasn't having any issue doing that. He was currently running at a 100% success rate in sticking a needle in my arm. It was the more refined task of finding an artery that was eluding him. The nurses were still being very attentive though. Closely observing the Master at work, still hoping to learn something other than how to apply a plaster over a ball of cotton wool.

Having needles stuck into your arm isn't *overly* painful although it can feel a bit *wincey* when the needles are wiggled. But it's surprising how quickly a sense of frustration can build in a patient when you realise the needle is off-target, and that the highly trained clinician will have to repeat the process.

Having assertively repositioned my arm flat on the bed, the Doc located another site on my left arm, in we go. Wiggle... jiggle ... and ... no. The Doc exhales, puts a ball of cotton wool over the needle and withdraws it. Just as one of the ever-prepared nurses is taping the fourth ball of cotton wool to my arm, Doc Swagger suddenly bursts out with, and I kid you not, 'This is doen' ma fackin' heed in.'

No sooner had he finished saying it, he looked at me, shocked, probably looking for my reaction and apologised. 'Jesus, I'm so sorry. I didnae mean you. Jus the situation. O' caus it's not you. Yev bin thru enough t'day.' It's worth remembering folks, 50% of all Doctors had to have finished in the bottom half of their medical class.

I played a very calm hand and told him not to worry about it. At that point, the non-student nurse stepped in and offered to try to get the needle in; an offer which he gladly accepted and of course, she succeeded, first time, back in the original arm. Far from being annoyed at being potentially upstaged by the nurse, he seemed quite relieved that, that phase was over; did what he had to do and finally inserted the guitar string up my ART. His chat was much more mellow whilst doing this and was asking about how I felt and what had happened. I was partway through my response when he interrupted, 'Oh it's you – ma mate is th' A&E consultant where the first took ye an' he phoned t' say tha' you were comin' over. Yours is th' ECG wi no real story on it.'

Yep, that's me – no real story.

You'd think that *not* having a load of shit written large across your ECG would feel like a good thing. But if that meant smart, well-trained, and super-experienced medical folk were left scratching their heads, then I wasn't feeling it.

My brother Mark and his wife Jayne came to visit later that afternoon. They'd driven 2 ½ hours from Cleethorpes. I'm sure the drive time had given them plenty of opportunity to think about what kind of a state I might be in, but they seemed if not impressed then relieved when they'd spent some time with me. Karina's sister, Sarah, and my Brother-in-law, Jus also visited. I can't recall too much about the visits, to be honest, but two, loosely related things do stand out.

Mark and Jayne were talking about something they had planned and were looking forward to; friends visiting or going away for the weekend. As if sharing some profound insight, I suddenly felt the need to offer, 'You absolutely enjoy yourselves! Do everything you can in life because this is it. I've been to the other side – and there's nothing there!'

I can appreciate, on reflection, although said with good intent, it was merely an unnecessary reminder for them of the awful events of the last few hours, so actually, that was a bit crap of me.

The other most significant conversation that afternoon was one that people often don't like talking about at the best of times, so it feels even worse at the worst of times. That topic being, my Last Will & Testament. Or more accurately, the lack thereof.

For years it'd been on the *to-do* list but like millions of others, we'd just never got around to it. To be fair to us, it wasn't morbidity or discussing death that had been the kicker of the can down the road. It was addressing the challenge of coming up with the best solution for our circumstances. We'd always felt it might not be that straightforward, given that in addition to the house and any bits and bobs of savings, we also had interests in two small businesses.

It was all a bit of a squishy Rubik's cube that needed proper discussions with proper experts to suggest proper solutions to help us make proper plans. This of course would have taken proper time, costing proper cash from a proper solicitor, so we'd just never got around to it. But circumstances had changed. Everyone around the CCU bed – as well as the person in it - all agreed, something was better than nothing. The most important thing was to avoid my estate being stuck in the limbo of Probate for months on end; should I ever end up becoming a more permanent resident on the other side.

The talk was, it was a given that it wouldn't be required, but at least it'd be there for peace of mind. Then, once all this was over, the whole thing could be revisited and sorted out properly, by a proper... you get the picture. As such, they agreed to go away and come up with a solution that evening.

Following the discussions about what to do with my Argentina '78 football sticker collection if I fell off my twig, I tried to offset some of this worry with a little bit of light humour. I opened with, 'Well, seeing as we're talking about life after Karl, it's good that you,' looking at my Bro, 'and you,' looking at Karina's Sister, 'are both here, as you can be witnesses to this.' There was a curiosity in the air, as to what was coming next. I then looked at Karina, held her hand and said, 'I don't want you to be lonely if anything happens to me. I just want you to be happy. Life's too short. So, after a short period of mourning of say, 36 years, if you wanted to be with someone else, I won't haunt you.'

OK, it probably sat more in the dark humour camp than light, but I was being sincere about the core message. The terms of the clause stating the moratorium, were of course, flexible.

I thought it was funny. Karina really didn't. To Karina, life without me wasn't even an option as a potential outcome. Just as it hadn't been, when she'd been beating the shit out of my chest, screaming, 'Not on my fucking watch,' earlier that day. Anything other than a positive outcome wasn't on the table. Perhaps recent events had compromised my filter but suffice to say, it didn't go down very well. Strange how you can be the source of so much worry and yet, be thought of as a total dick, at the same time.

Three of them spent most of that night researching, downloading templates, editing, drafting, and redrafting a Will; eventually getting to a bunch of words, in a sequence that made sense for our requirements. Although she had her practical boots on, this must have been quite tough for Karina. She would have been repeatedly told this was just an academic exercise; a belt 'n' braces process; an item of housekeeping admin which had no relevance whatsoever. And yet, there she was, having to pull it all together as an act of necessity, without me being there. Even with the others there, that must have been a lonely and unpleasant experience.

The rest of the day and evening was positively uneventful for me, thankfully. Not so for everyone around me. Alarms were sounding. A Crash Team was needed for one. Sobbing came from a room somewhere on the other side – I never did find out why. I didn't particularly want to know. There was a permanent air of being in a *high state of alert*. Unsurprising, given the poorliness that enveloped the place. Even a nurse broke her thumb and disappeared to X-ray.

I was anchoring my positivity to the fact that I was feeling generally OK, but it was challenged by almost everything I was hearing and seeing. It was difficult to keep darker thoughts from gaining traction in my mind. And by gaining more traction I mean, whenever I saw a really poorly person in that CCU, I couldn't help wondering, is that suddenly going to be me?

# 16

## 8 Percent

*"When we're no longer able to change a situation,
we are challenged to change ourselves."*
**Viktor Frankl**

The following day, at 9am, I was shocked as Gordon approached
my bed. Not shocked at him coming to visit me as I'd imagined he
would at some point. The shock lay in how he looked. I'd only ever
seen him as the epitome of chilled and calm; a vision of reassurance
and quiet confidence in his delivery and assessment. He was a Cardiologist. This was CCU. This was his patch, his manor. Each member
of staff cheerily greeted him as he passed them by and he replied, but
in a somewhat subdued and distant manner. There was no under-
stated presence of a man at the top of his game. No air of confidence
as an apex operator.

The person approaching me was ashen-faced, visibly upset and
stunned. I'd even go as far as to say he looked humble as he pulled up
a chair. Which was saying something because I'd never seen him look
*unhumble* if that's a word. But the Doctor who'd never been short of
calming tones was now almost at a loss for words. Doctor Sting had
become Doctor Stung. This was a man who'd clearly had very little
sleep.

He opened by expressing how sorry he was to see me back in hospital but on the flip side, how thankful he was, that I was in CCU.

Unusual angle, I thought.

There was a brief conversation; he asked me how I'd felt after leaving hospital; had I felt any pain or warning signs prior to the cardiac arrest. He was as deadpan as a deceased pan could be. There was no twinkle or shine in his eyes. They were fixed on me as though analysing dire information for the first time.

He asked how I was currently feeling, and I was honest, in that, I was mostly feeling OK apart from the intense pain everywhere across the front of my ribs. He was very quick to respond, 'Yes... well the compression pains will completely disappear once we've cut through your sternum. Believe me, they'll no longer be a concern for you.'

Hmmm. Relief *and* trepidation delivered in one breath. Then started probably the most eye-opening conversation of my life.

Gordon started telling me how phenomenally well Karina had done, not just in her CPR but in keeping her shit (my word, not his) together. Delivering CPR correctly and successfully was an incredibly difficult thing to do. He enquired as to whether she had any medical background or emergency services training, to which I said she hadn't. This he found even more incredible and went on to explain why.

'It's not like in the movies or on TV, where someone drowns or has a heart attack, followed by a bit of chest-pounding and suddenly the patient splutters, coughs and sits up. I wish it was, but it hardly ever happens that way.' He underlined the point. 'Bystander CPR success rate is incredibly low – about 8%.'

I was numbed. It was all coming together now: the Paramedic saying that in 16 years he'd never seen a response like it; the other Paramedic telling me I'd had a very fortunate outcome; the A&E Consultant describing Karina's actions as 'remarkable' and assuming she was medically trained. 8%? My overriding thought was, 'I'm never that lucky.' If there was a bowl of 100 balls and 8 of them could win me £1million, there's no way I'd ever pull out a winner.

Gordon continued. 'I mean, we call it Bystander CPR - that just means out of hospital CPR. This was your wife, not a random stranger in the street, so she had a vested interest. She might have put a bit more into it,' he gave a little smile. 'But then often people just go to pieces when it's a loved one, so sometimes you're better off if it's a genuine stranger.'

I have no idea how I responded to this information; except I was stunned at the number. 8%. It was difficult to process what I was hearing and that it applied to me, but he hadn't finished.

'Even in hospital with trained medical staff, all the necessary equipment and all the right medicines and oxygen on hand, CPR success rate is still low; barely double that. 16% if we're lucky.'

I was staggered. If I'd been asked, I'd have thought it'd be somewhere around 70-80% in hospital and maybe 60% anywhere else. Gordon wasn't finished though. 'And then of those 8%, maybe 50% could have some sort of brain damage.'

Brain damage? Shit! A thought flashed across my mind and began to form on my lips. Gordon read it before the words had even hit the airwaves.

'And if you're wondering if you've got brain damage, the fact that you're even wondering it would tell me you haven't. When I say brain damage, some people are left with life-changing issues and will never work or really do anything for themselves, again. Others might have symptoms similar to a mild stroke, which maybe they eventually recover from.' There was a brief pause. 'You really do owe an awful lot to your wife.'

I was just nodding numbly, barely able to comprehend the narrowness of the window I'd climbed through when he suddenly adopted a different tone for a different line of conversation.

'But,' he said firmly, looking me straight in the eyes, 'we clearly have to wonder about the decision to discharge you on Tuesday. To have a cardiac arrest 18 hours after being discharged from, effectively a three-week spell in hospital for cardiac issues, should *not* have happened. I'm really very, very sorry. For what you went through and for what Karina had to go through. I want to re-assure you that we will learn from this and will be reviewing our processes and protocols.'

This was an interesting juncture in the conversation, and I sensed that he felt, where it went from there, was largely down to me. To put it bluntly, I could have gone nuclear about what had happened. But at that very point in time, 9am on Thursday 9th May, my clarity of thought and belief were as crystal clear and aligned as they'd ever been in my life. I was looking at life from the square I was standing on and through a purely selfish lens. And when I say selfish, I mean selfish in its absolutely literal sense.

All I wanted to do, was to move on from that square, as quickly and successfully as possible. My focus and energy were on nothing else. The last thing on my mind was retribution, of any type. These people were exceptionally talented at their jobs – I needed them to channel everything they could, into fixing me. I needed Team Pezza at the top of its game. If they felt *they owed me*, even just a little, that would be welcome, but the reality was, I was entirely in their healing hands.

By way of confirmation of where I stood on the matter, I said, 'Gordon, I'm not holding anyone to blame or pointing any fingers. I've got no axe to grind on the decision. I just want to get myself fixed and back to a normal, active life.' He was a decent man and he clearly cared about his patients. Although, it was strange that for once, I was in the unusual position of providing reassurance to him. Or so it felt.

Now it was clear the elephant in the room had been addressed and it wasn't going to cause a stampede, matters moved on to practical issues. I was told that providing Mr D could get the surgical team together he wanted, it was looking like my operation would take place on Saturday morning.

I like a man who's fussy about who he works with. It says a lot about his character and expectations, and given his surgical reputation, it says a lot about his team's character too.

48 hours. That's all I had to wait for the Grand Opening. I was so relieved. Again, strange that the prospect of being cut open and having your heart stopped and sliced, would bring such relief and positivity. But that's the thing, it's not the cutting and slicing that brings the relief and positivity. That's just the process. It's the end result that brings the relief and the positivity. The normality and opportunity for a fully active life. But you can't have one without going through the other. You've just got to survive the other.

Prior to the conversation with Gordon, if I'd had to put recent events on a *just how bad was this?* scale, I would've been somewhere around the *that could've been a lot worse* mark. This was the first time it'd crossed my mind that there wasn't that much wiggle room left for things to have gone much worse. I was beginning to feel like I'd dodged a bullet. Even then, I wasn't sure *dodged* was exactly the right word, as it dawned on me that, for a short while, I'd been dead.

Usually, death is associated with the point from which there is no return. Although apparently, medically speaking, death is a biological process, which can take place at different rates throughout different parts of the body. However, it's generally accepted that, if your heart stops beating and you're no longer breathing, then you're dead. Sometimes the heart can be restarted – and then you're not dead. I'm not sure if there's a word for the bit in between - if you're one of the lucky 8% to have the bit in between.

I was far, far away from coming to terms with what all this meant and what I felt about it. In fact, it'd barely scratched the surface of my consciousness. I knew I'd have to address it at some point. I also knew it'd take up a lot of energy doing so. Likewise, I'd only really had a topline conversation with Karina about what had happened during those few minutes when I was off the grid. I had so many questions and there was so much I wanted to know about that time in between being alive and being alive. But l also knew processing all that stuff would be emotionally and physically draining. For both of us.

I'd just been told there were 48 hours until my operation. Notwithstanding that the procedure was carried out in many hospitals around the country, many times a day, with an incredibly high success rate and - initially more importantly - survival rate, there was no getting away from it. This was a major operation with a great many risks. Possibly more so now, given my heart had just undergone the trauma of an arrest followed by a re-start. Whilst I had every faith in the lead surgeon and his team, I was under no illusion there were any guarantees.

As such, I made a conscious decision to park my need for deeper enquiries with Karina, as well as avoiding thinking too much about how close I'd come to the point of no return. And what that would've meant, for my family and everything else in my entire life. I decided my focus needed to be on preparing for the operation. All my energy had to go into that. And by not thinking about the near-miss of finality, I could hopefully avoid or at least minimise distress, stress and becoming a mess. All of which would help keep a lid on blood pressure, heart rate and to some degree heart rhythm. My inner voice even went so far as to tell me that reflecting, might just be a waste of time anyway. If I didn't survive the operation, what would've been the point of over-analysing recent events? I might as well wait and see if there even was an *after the operation,* and revisit events then. There would be plenty of time to do so if there was.

I'm paraphrasing this conversation with my inner bully/mentor/self but that was pretty much the gist of it. To be fair, I was grateful to that little voice. Despite wanting answers and time to reflect, the voice was quite right. It was all irrelevant unless I passed *Go* again, so my plan made complete sense to me. We all have that little voice, don't we? You know the one. The one that gives you a completely honest precis on your own thoughts and behaviours, regardless of what spin you wished you could put on something. It's more than just your conscience. It's that and your gut and millions of years of evolution, all rolled up into one internal mouthpiece, giving you direction based loosely on the principles of fight, flight, or freeze. Mine was telling me to fight but was being selective about on which fronts.

I'm not sure if this is the right time to bring it up but I might as well, as you've possibly already been wondering about it. So many people have asked me about it so I'll share it with you too. Within a day of 8th May, once people had heard the news, had enquired as to how I was and had established that I was broadly stable, the next most asked question was some variant of, 'So what's it like to be dead?'

For me, this is a very straightforward answer, although I'm aware there's the potential for it to become complicated. To recap, I can remember talking with Karina, but with absolutely no fade-to-titles sequence. The next thing I knew, there is a fade-in, firstly by touch, then by sound, followed by sight, but as for what was in between.

Nothing.

I can't even say blackness, because that suggests I was conscious of myself and the complete lack of stimuli around me. Not true. It was simply a badly edited experience starting from a rough-cut mid-frame to a fade-in to what felt like a completely different movie.

I had no concept of time, movement, vision, or hearing. There were no dream sequences, nightmares, or musical interludes. I had no sense of self-awareness, emotion, or anything remotely like an out-of-body experience.

Equally, there were no bright lights, illuminated ascending stairways, grand entranceways to gated communities, Saintly bureaucrats armed with clipboards or winged cherubs, hovering like drones. Likewise, there were no descending stairways, fiery glows, demonic welcome parties, or a sense of unbearable heat.

There was no gathering of deceased family members and friends, or Elvis, come to that. Not even any alien life forms waiting to take the soul of one of the toys from their experimental hobby, back to the Mothership.

All disappointingly, not the case. We go through life, not knowing for sure, if there's anything at all to look forward to, after death. Some hope, some don't. Some believe, some debunk. Even as an atheist I'd love to have been able to have discovered something - anything, that suggested there was more than just a full-stop after our final breath. But I didn't.

But here's where potentially it can become complicated. Some people may suggest, as I'm here, living and breathing, that I didn't actually die and therefore cannot truthfully report from the other side. I can understand this thinking but looking at the facts, I wasn't breathing, and my heart had stopped beating. Although there is the potential to reverse this scenario within a certain limited time frame, you'd have to ask, reverse from what?

Secondly – and theologically I completely accept this point – my belief system may have had a lot to do with my experience. As I say, I'm an atheist. I don't believe in a Creator, the whole concept of an afterlife or the notion of Heaven. Now if I'm wrong, and those things do exist, perhaps the afterlife is administered in such a way that us non-believers don't get to see it. I mean, if there is a God, and this Creator is as kind and benevolent as 3000 different global religions believe, (childhood cancer, genocides, and Jimmy Saville aside) then this would make sense. Of course, non-believers like me, wouldn't get to see any of the eternal good stuff. What kind of despot psycho would show me that? That would be like saying, 'This is what you could have won,' as I slept rough against the outer wall of the Kingdom of Heaven for all eternity.

Or maybe there's yet another alternative. Perhaps everyone is initially corralled into some kind of holding pen; a heavenly sensory deprivation chamber, until it's decided whether we're staying for the long term or being claimed back. Like an item of lost property.

I have no idea how the afterlife, if there is such a thing, operates. All I can say is, I've seen nothing to change my mind, but equally, I'm none the wiser. I'm a pro-faith atheist. I don't believe but I recognise the right of others to do so. Believe in whatever you want. Just don't make it a mission to convince others that your way of thinking – yay or nay – is undeniably true. It isn't and never can be. Besides, life here is far too short and apparently, it can be taken away, randomly at any given second. Here endeth the lesson. Amen.

Later that morning, Karina, Sarah, Mark and Jayne brought the finished Will in, which I scanned through and duly signed, barely taking the contents in. I suppose part of me felt, whatever was mine was Karina's anyway and if I were to become the ex-tenant of this mortal coil, then it'd be someone else's knot to untangle, should my Last Will & Testament generate said knot.

'Oooo ... you selfish bastard,' I hear the gallery cry.

Well... yea, I guess so – but in that truest of senses. As I say, I'd already recognised that I couldn't afford to give up much headspace to anything other than trying to keep myself on an even keel, ahead of entering the operating theatre. After that, it was over to the surgeons. I'd have done my bit, but by that point, I'd be in their hands completely – and literally.

It does sound quite strange with hindsight, but I never overly worried about not making it to the operation or not getting through it. On the contrary, I was totally aware that either of those things could potentially happen. My head wasn't in the sand; I wasn't in denial. I got it. But equally, I recognised there was so little I could control, why waste energy worrying about that lack of control and the *what-ifs*? I parked everything, literally everything I regarded as non-essential, including negative thoughts and to some extent, some degree of emotion.

As I write this I wonder if this is some sort of Survivor Bias coming through, but I don't think so. I'm not saying I kept a lid on everything all the time, but I recognised the futility of investing in negative thoughts, worrying, and playing out future scenarios in which I'd be no longer present. So, I chose not to. It was possibly the most focused I'd ever been in my entire life.

So, the Will was signed, and I knew that once all this was over, we'd get it all sorted out properly.

I can honestly say I haven't seen that piece of paper since, and I have absolutely no idea where it is.

# 17

# What Are The Chances?

*"Your body can stand almost anything.*
*It's your mind you have to convince."*
**Unknown**

Later that afternoon, a Doctor I'd not met before arrived to carry out an ultrasound scan. I was pretty relaxed until she dropped the bombshell; it may now be Tuesday when they operate.

Déjà vu... here we go again. Mission creep.

Having just explained how I'd managed to filter out most of the emotions centred around fear and worry, dealing with frustration proved a little more challenging. Well initially, certainly, as I made no attempt to deploy my poker face. She probably also saw it on her screen as my heart advanced towards fight mode. She tried to pull it back. Saturday was still the preferred date apparently, but Mr D was having difficulties getting all his preferred team together for then.

This was so tough to hear. Saturday was big match day and I was already well into my mental preparation. I'd been on top of it. Confident in the surgeon and focused on the countdown to a new, stronger, healthier, stage in my life. Tuesday was an additional three days. I really didn't want to wait that long. Sure, there was a huge element of fear in what the waiting may do to my already underperforming heart, but the thought of standing down and having to reset myself mentally was the biggest blow. I was ready, there and then. If they'd said, 'You're being bumped up, it's in six hours,' I'd have been over the moon. By then, I just wanted the solution to the problem, and as soon as possible. Being told it could be five days away drained the energy away from me. Exactly what I had been focused on avoiding.

This poor Doctor had just thought she was having a gentle conversation; some medical small talk whilst she carried out a fairly routine scan. She couldn't have anticipated that she'd be delivering possibly the second shittest news of the week. Possibly of my life, at that point. The operation wasn't merely my gateway to moving on from the last few years and getting back to an active life. It was about survival. Moving it further away, felt like the risks would be multiplying and my mental resilience would be stretched more thinly.

The obs continued every few hours; blood samples were taken; the Californian carafes were taken away; food came and went as did my close family visitors. But all the time I was thinking about the operation date. By Thursday evening I still hadn't heard any news. Although, I don't know how, by then I'd managed to flick a mental switch. I knew I'd find out for sure the following day. And I decided I should continue preparing for a Saturday operation, so when the news came, if Saturday was D-Day, then I was still mentally on track.

Decision made. I felt in control once again and it was the obvious position to take. I wondered why it had taken me so long to get my head around it and why I'd allowed it to wind me up so much. Sometimes, you just get tired and fed up worrying. I was rewarded with a really good night's sleep, which was unusual considering where my bed was located.

My positivity had stayed with me overnight and I woke the next day – Friday 10th May feeling vaguely excited. There was going to be significant movement over the next few hours. I'd find out for definite if my operation would be taking place the following day and if so, there'd be a fair bit of pre-op prep, I imagined. If it was to be Tuesday, then I'd prepared myself for that too and had decided to break the days down into thirds again and to fill each one with something: visitor chat/reading/sleeping/Netflix-ing/responding to the backlog of messages building up on text/WhatsApp/Messenger/email/voicemail. I'd slipped into radio silence on all channels, and I needed to address that.

I went on to Facebook to see what was going on in the world. I'm not sure why really. I had no intention of posting anything. I hardly ever posted. Maybe a handful of times a year. It was never my intention to broadcast my situation on FB or any other social media. The thought of generating the attention and then needing to respond to it never appealed to me. I know it would for many on there. For many, social media is just a massive flag to wave shouting, 'Look at me! Look at me!' for whatever spurious reason. Or worse, to peddle their *Outrage Porn*. It's really not me. I was never even sure why I had an account. Probably to satisfy the voyeur in me by looking at other people's flag-waving. And to take the piss out of sad, attention-seeking, dick-drips who habitually lick their wounds of offence, so publicly. (Which can be quite fun, I suppose.)

So, for whatever reason, I went onto FB and quite quickly a narrative was beginning to appear. Something had obviously happened to someone I'd gone to school with. Something not good. Something terminal.

There was an outpouring of condolences, shock, comforting memes, grief, heavenly themes, poignant quotations, and general talk of another star in the sky and a new angel in paradise.

If you'd known this guy (let's call him Danny) growing up in school in the 1970s and 80s, very few would have put the word *angel* in the same sentence as his name.

Danny habitually had skirmishes with teachers, kids in school, kids from other schools after school, and kids and referees in school football matches. He could pick a fight with his own shadow. He left school at 15. Like us, he was supposed to have left at 16, but he walked out to join his brothers' building firm. From memory, the school didn't try too hard to stop him.

His choice of career came as no surprise. At 15, Danny was more man than most men we knew. After sports lessons, we'd all have to take a communal shower, so everything was on show. At age 12, when some of us were still counting hairs on one hand, Danny had cultivated a full privet hedge and could have taken the lead role in a porn film. He wasn't shy about pointing these differences out to us, either.

But for all his skirmishes, I'd always got on with him and had never fallen foul of any rage he'd vented. The same went for most of my mates. In fact, there was a time both in junior school and in our early pub-going careers, when Danny was a regular member of the gang. Always good for a laugh and always good for a story.

And now, it appeared that suddenly, something dreadful had happened to him. I text my best mate from Cleethorpes and someone else who'd grown up with him through school and our early pub days. It appeared he'd had a motorbike crash on a motorway in the early hours of 8th May. By the time my heart had stopped beating on that same day, Danny was already dead. Two lads from the same class through school, on the same day. What were the chances? And yet I was still here.

I couldn't remember the last time I'd seen him or physically spoken with him, but it hit me hard. The finality of death. Of mortality. Those outpourings of memes and quotes and messages of shock and sympathy could have been for me. I'd been so close to that happening, and that would have closed the door. The Paramedics would have been gutted I'm sure but would have had to move on to their next job. But my whole world and that of my family would have been broken forever.

To be one of the lucky 8 percenters was one thing, but then hearing about Danny losing his life on the same day I'd crossed the abys and returned, really brought everything into the sharpest of all imaginable focus. Reading through the posts was like holding a mirror up to my life; to what so nearly could have been. Having felt so confidently in control of my emotions, I suddenly felt quite afraid and vulnerable. Shocked at what had happened to me only 48 hours before. I really, desperately wanted this operation to take place the following day. I needed it to. Suddenly, the thought of waiting until Tuesday felt a bridge too far. That time had become my enemy.

Shortly after 9am, Mr D entered the room and approached my bed. I was about to get my answer.

'So, you've probably heard your operation may have been postponed to Tuesday?'

Here we go. 'Yes, I have.'

'Well, I still want to go ahead tomorrow.'

My face lit up. 'That's great news!'

'That's not usually the reaction I get when I tell people that.'

I started to tell him about my school friend. He couldn't have been less interested.

'However, there's a caveat,' he said. 'The only thing that may bump it is if we get an emergency heart transplant come in, but we'll know whether that's the case by about 7 o'clock tonight.'

*DAMN!!* I was almost totally over the line but there was *still* the possibility it may not happen... my face must have said, as he then followed up with, 'But it's unlikely.'

He then went through the consent form with me, explaining what the procedure would entail; all the risks, including death, which statistically was about 1-2%. I thought 1 in 50 was quite high, but he explained that most patients were much older than me and had many co-morbidities which can complicate things.

Not that I had any choice in the matter. *Not* having the procedure wasn't an option. That path would guarantee an early exit. And this really wasn't a buyer's market. There wasn't the option of saying, 'Oooo – I don't really fancy those odds. Have you got anything that does the same sort of thing but with less chance of my family having to wear black in a few weeks?'

I duly signed the consent form.

He also pointed out there was a small chance the operation could cause an issue with my heart rate some time afterwards, which could result in a pacemaker being fitted.

'What kind of chance?' I asked.

'Less than 1 in 20,' he replied.

So that's 20 balls, with one loser... possible... but still unlikely.

'No problem,' I decided, and signed the separate confirmation of understanding.

And then there was a final topic for discussion. I was due to have a repair to my Mitral Valve; one of Mr D's many areas of expertise. So much so, that when a Doctor the previous day, learned who'd be carrying out the procedure, they reassuringly referred to him as *Mr Mitral*.

Mr D advised that he foresaw no complications to this repair. However, if once *inside,* he discovered hitherto unknown issues, or that a repair really wouldn't do the job, then the sensible thing would be to replace the valve, there and then. There'd be no point in doing everything else only to come back and be opened up for a second time to have the valve replaced.

I completely agreed. Where do I sign?

Apparently, it wasn't that straightforward. I had to decide as to whether I'd want an artificial or tissue valve as the replacement. *Should* the need arise. Which of course he kept stressing, he felt would be extremely unlikely. And by the way, by *tissue*, they mean a valve from a pig's heart or crafted from the heart sack of a cow. That in itself is enough to put some people off this option, but I had no issue with this aspect whatsoever.

Not having specialised in heart valve replacement at any point in my life, I knew not one single thing about either option, so asked the guy in front of me, which he would recommend. Surprisingly, he couldn't offer any opinion. By *couldn't*, he meant, he wasn't ethically allowed to direct a patient to either option. This decision had to be entirely down to patient choice as there were pros and cons associated with each solution. What he was able to do though, was go through those.

Again, invoking my frequently used caveat; the following words are my own to briefly summarise the differences between the two options, as each option potentially offered a greatly different onward journey and user experience. Apologies to any cardiac heavyweights or manufacturers of replacement valves, reading this if I've oversimplified things. But just imagine how it felt to be the patient going through this, because believe me, in that position, we want it as simple as possible.

The artificial or mechanical valve would more than likely last for the rest of my life. Whereas the tissue valve may need to be replaced after 10-12 years, but maybe as soon as seven years, or it may last as long as 15-20 years. But assuming I lived an average lifetime, it would eventually need to be replaced, which would potentially but not necessarily, mean another open-heart procedure.

Hmmm... having to go through this process again, didn't endear me to the tissue option. Round one to the mechanical valve.

However, the mechanical valve increased the likelihood of clots forming which, as we know, is not something to aspire to. As such, a mechanical valve would mean a lifetime of being on a drug called Warfarin. Warfarin is a bit of a pain as I'd have to be tested every few weeks to make sure my blood INR levels (the measure for how long it takes to clot) didn't fluctuate outside a certain range. I knew from my Mum being on Warfarin that it's a sensitive little soul. Your INR can be influenced by so many factors such as other medications, diet, tea, coffee, rolling your eyes, a strong easterly wind and alcohol consumption. (Not all of this is true.)

The tissue option would require my usual blood thinners which didn't require constant monitoring. Round 2 to the tissue option.

Another factor to consider was that many patients report they can hear and feel their artificial valves closing. To some, this can be very distressing. In fact, I recalled during my earlier stay on the cardio-thoracic ward, a guy in our bay was so distressed that after about a week, he had it removed, and a tissue valve put in. How awful. The thought of hearing the clunk, clunk, clunk of the valve would just be a constant reminder of what had happened and would probably drive me insane.

Round 3 to the tissue option.

But really, I still only knew what I'd just been told about them. Typically for me, I felt I had to do more research so asked for more time. I also asked if there was any more information he could give me. He said not, except to say that such rapid advances were being made in this area that all kinds of possibilities would be available in the near future. No rush - I could let them know first thing in the morning, as they had plenty of both options in stock. Which came across as a bit weird. Like having loads of car parts in a garage. But then I suppose that's exactly what it's like.

So that was my mission for the rest of the day. To research and decide on whether to have a valve that would last the rest of my life but would scare the shit out of the passenger next to me in the quiet carriage on the train to London. Along with a lifetime on a pain-in-the-arse drug with a mind of its own. Or the quieter, easier to manage option, which could require another major operation when I'm older, weaker, less resilient to infection and possibly dealing with other health issues, that may or may not have come along by then.

And this, don't forget, was all on the *off chance* of being needed. I was to choose between actual solutions to a hypothetical problem.

By mid-afternoon, I'd decided. I'd decided that the day-to-day experience was more important to me and that being happy during that time would encourage and help me to stay healthy. And by being healthy, I'd still be in a good position to face a major operation 7 to 15 or even 20 years down the line.

It felt really positive to have made the decision and that I could rationalise it, even though the whole decision-making process would hopefully, or rather was more likely to have been a completely academic exercise.

Whether the process ultimately proved to be a waste of time or not, the single biggest benefit to me on Friday 10th May, was that it had occupied my mind; taken it off the death of a school pal and had helped to run down the clock. It would have been about 3 o'clock by then. Which meant I only had about four hours to go before I'd be given the green light confirming the game was most definitely afoot.

# 18

## The Anaesthetist

*"Sometimes when you're in a dark place you think you've been buried, but you've actually been planted."*
**Christine Caine**

By the time 7pm arrived, I was almost giddy there'd been no message of postponement due to an unknown tragedy elsewhere. Someone, somewhere else, was still desperate for a donor heart and equally, someone somewhere else was still very much alive. This was very good news for two out of three of us. Of course, I had the time of 7pm in my head as a fixed finish line, beyond which, we were into Thunderbirds Are Go! territory. But just as no one had told me it was off, no one had confirmed it was on, either.

I asked a nurse, how I'd find out if it was definitely on and she replied they assumed the operation would be taking place unless they heard otherwise. But an Anaesthetist would need to chat with me first anyway. So, if that happened, that would be my answer.

*Assumed*? I really didn't like that word. By that stage, I wanted hard, black and white, immovable facts. I was about to test her customer service skills when suddenly, *The Shopkeeper* appeared. Or more accurately, the Anaesthetist.

He was quite a big guy, tall and full-bodied; probably early 40s and a little gruff sounding. If you'd seen him on the street, you'd probably have guessed at several other career options before getting to Anaesthetist. *Gangster* was the first that sprang to my mind. Not that I was questioning his ability to do his job. If he was on Mr D's team, I was more than happy not to judge the medical book by its cover. But most importantly, the fact he was by my bed, meant Operation Pezza had been green-lighted for the following day. The countdown could begin, and I had an overwhelming sense of relief. Out came the forms and the questions began.

Once we'd established I had no other medical conditions, allergies and hadn't reacted badly to anaesthetic in the past, we were done. Just as he was wrapping up, he asked if anyone had discussed the kind of valve I'd want, if a repair wasn't feasible. I explained Mr D, had brought this up and after lengthy research, I'd decided on the tissue option, but I could let him know in the morning.

Looking at me earnestly he asked, 'Are you sure about that?'

'Yes definitely. He only asked this morning but said I could let him know first thing tomorrow before I go in.'

'No, I mean about choosing the tissue valve,' he replied.

His response took me a bit by surprise. Firstly because I'd been asked to make the decision independently. I'd done so and felt I could justify this decision logically and emotionally, so why was this guy challenging it?

But secondly, Mr Soprano here, was the Anaesthetist, so what the hell had it got to do with him, anyway? Wasn't he just there to knock me out and keep me knocked out for the duration of the operation and a little bit afterwards? (I know. I know. Apologies to any Anaesthetists, for the oversimplified job description.)

I confirmed I was sure and that I'd made up my mind. But he wasn't leaving anything to chance.

'I'm not so sure that's a good decision. The tissue valve will need replacing in a few years and it'll mean another big operation. It's not an easy thing to perform or to go through. You might end up having to have an artificial valve put in at that point anyway. And don't forget, you'll probably be weaker; you might have other medical issues going on by then which could complicate things. Your heart might even be damaged. I really wouldn't advise it.'

What happened to not being ethically allowed to direct the patient? Did this guy have a side hustle in mechanical valves? I mean, there was a lot of speculation in there. A lot of *what-ifs* and *could bes*. Which, yes, possibly could conspire to create the scenario he'd described. Possibly.

But what would be a *definite* if I went down the artificial route, was that I'd be clunking around like The Tin Man for the rest of my life, whilst having to pop a drug with the sensitivity of a Premiership Footballer.

He signed off the conversation with, 'It's your choice. It wouldn't be mine.'

This is the caveat universally accepted as, *don't say I didn't warn you when it all goes tits up*, which is lovely to hear less than three days after a cardiac arrest and the evening before you go into a lengthy, life-enabling operation.

It goes without saying, this man hadn't pushed himself to the top of my Christmas card list, but I was keen not to show it. I still needed him at the top of his game, and I wasn't going out of my way to piss off the guy injecting the juice. Mr Chippy stayed in his box.

A little later, a nurse came over to run through the timings of the pre-op schedule. Last solids at 10pm, thereafter a lemon flavoured liquid meal which would be repeated at about 7am. Mr D would visit me around 8am, Karina could visit from about 8:30 and they would be waiting for the call to transfer me to the Theatre from 9am. Then the biggy – and I'd been wondering when it would be coming – *The Shave*.

As I say, I'd heard it so many times before whilst on the ward – the pre-match prep. The high-pitched buzz from behind pulled curtains, signalling that a nurse was helping a chap part with his bodily down. Who was holding what, I'd shuddered to imagine, but it had become symbolic of the imminence of even sharper instruments coming into contact with the body. The final resignation of what was shortly to come.

The nurse was stood there with the cordless electric razor, and I was expecting her to reach for the curtains, but to my mild surprise, she asked if I'd prefer to shave myself in the privacy of the shower room? If so, she could grab a wheelchair and push me there. I seized the opportunity with all my limbs. I'd initially thought it was decent of her to allow her patient to retain as much dignity as possible. But with hindsight, having to shave around some older bloke's tackle probably didn't feature in her *top 100 things I love about my job* list.

I was wheeled to the shower room and asked to shave off everything from my neck down to both ankles and my left arm. This worried me greatly. I knew they were hoping to use the internal Mammary Artery but if there was an issue, they'd harvest one from my leg. But apparently, in case there were complications on the complications, they'd need the option of my other leg. The arm, I think, was just for fun. The thought of having wounds to heal in both legs as well as my chest just filled me with dread. So many more opportunities for infection.

I was told to take as long as I needed and to pull one of the many emergency chords dotted around the shower room when I was ready to be wheeled back to my bed. The nurse shut the door and I locked it. It was just me and the razor. I switched it on, and its high-pitched buzz signalled the start of what I hoped would ultimately be a positive if not lengthy process of getting me back to a normal, hospital-free life.

Shaving with an electric razor is not, by any stretch, a painful process. But as I set about slowly removing my body hair so that the surgeons could have their way with me, I had a sense of trepidation. And for the first time on this whole journey, I became aware of another feeling, one that I rarely felt. I began to feel a bit sorry for myself.

It's ridiculous really, but I did. Cardiac arrest and imminent heart bypass withstanding, I was in far better shape with a far better prognosis than so many other people both inside and outside the hospital. I absolutely knew this and believed it, so it was a confusing feeling. I wasn't sure why I had this sudden sense of self-pity. But alone, in that room, having to shave my body, I don't know; there was a sense of foreboding. Maybe even a sense that it was degrading. It was difficult to get my head around why I felt that way. It's not as if it was a punishment shaving, designed to strip me of my worth. It was purely to help the surgeons do their work. To make the process more efficient. But still, that's how I felt. Sad and a bit lonely.

I took ages; much longer than was necessary. I didn't want to rush and make a hack job of it. I made sure I was as smooth as a baby's bot. I didn't want to wake up and discover that they'd pulled the operation due to my poor manscaping skills.

I even tidied up my beard. Somewhere at the back of my mind, I knew I didn't want to be laying there looking scruffy for Karina if the worst happened whilst I was on the table.

Once I was back in my bed, shaved and showered, I tucked into the lemon energy drink and picked up my phone. I was absolutely resigned to having the bypass. Not having it, wasn't an option. Life wouldn't have lasted much longer without it, so it wasn't exactly the *rock and a hard place* scenario. But the operation wasn't without risks and as frequently as these procedures are carried out, not everyone makes it. If they did, there wouldn't be as much fuss made over the consent form.

As such, I felt the absolute need to send some texts to a small group of family and friends. Without wanting to sound too dramatic, I wanted to make sure some key people had received a text or texts from me that could, if needed be, be interpreted as a goodbye. Or at the very least, as a decent sign off; without even approaching saying a goodbye. It's a fine line. Once I'd done this, I felt much more relaxed. I knew the operation was my only way out, and that it was happening the following day, was only a good thing. On the back of this, I went to sleep quite quickly and once again, slept remarkably well, all things considered.

The next day, I woke well before the need to be woken, around 6am and replied to a bunch of texts I'd received overnight in response to mine. So much for final texts. I felt surprisingly at ease with my situation. I was more than prepared for it, as I slipped into my open-backed gown and put my tissue-thin nappy pants on. They really need to work on their Spring range for patients.

Mr D arrived in good time. I'd only ever seen him in a suit, but he was already in his scrubs. His battle dress. They were a nice blue colour, but I expected I'd soon be changing that. He was there to check I was OK, composed and not shaking like a dog shitting Lego bricks. Naturally, the main topic of conversation was about the valve choice: *only if absolutely necessary, of course.*

I gave him my choice of the tissue valve and with an enthusiasm I hadn't seen before in this usually quiet and conservative man, he almost blurted out, 'That's exactly the decision I would have made!!'

Wow! If only he'd shared his preference when I first asked. I would have been freed up to watch the whole of Fleabag on iPlayer.

He asked if I had any concerns. On the one hand, I could have said, 'How long have you got?' but the reality was, we were where we were. I said that I hadn't, although having seen patients on the ward, I wasn't looking forward to the immediate few days after the operation. He looked a bit surprised. 'Oh, you won't feel any pain or discomfort. Your ribcage will be totally wired together so won't be going anywhere and you'll be so full of morphine you'll mostly be asleep.'

He made my part in it sound so easy. I almost believed him.

Off he went and Karina arrived. We were only scheduled to have 30 minutes before I was called, so I gave her a quick update on the Anaesthetist looking to expand his job description, Mr D's visit and of course my new shaven haven look.

During this new spell in hospital, we'd completely downplayed the reason why I'd gone back in so suddenly, to the kids. On that Wednesday, one had been at school and the other had been at College. We didn't want to worry them or add to their exam stress by sharing what had happened, so had told them I'd felt some pain in my chest and we'd gone in to get it checked out. (Technically not a lie, although the chest pain only began after the compressions, the two electric shocks and I'd regained consciousness). On the back of that, the Doctors had decided to bring the operation forward (again, not really a lie). As such, they'd only visited once since Wednesday and we'd been trying to downplay the operation being that day, but they obviously had their concerns. They weren't stupid and it's so easy to find answers on Google. Not necessarily the right answers, but answers, nonetheless.

You can argue whether it was the right or wrong approach - and we had done, at length - but it was done with the best of intentions to protect them. We'd 'fess up at some point in the near future to correct this economical truth.

Just after 9am, I swapped my bed for a wheelchair and was taken through a labyrinth of corridors. Karina joined me as far as the doors to the whole Theatre area. We kissed goodbye and I was taken through double doors into the world where the major medical stuff really happens. I was more than a little afraid when I left Karina but tried not to show it, for her and for me. I knew I had to go through with it – it was the *getting* through it, that was the unknown. We turned through another set of double doors and I was in the operating theatre.

It was a hive of activity. People were moving around with a sense of urgency. Once again, I was asked to lay on a raised bed I had to climb up, to get onto. A bed that was far too narrow for me, until the armrests were slid in. The heated blanket was placed on top of me, which was nice, but I still felt a little cold. Maybe it was just a nervous shiver. Something was being connected to the cannula in my left arm, a blood pressure cuff was being applied to my other arm, electrodes were stuck in various locations; I was asked a few questions, name, DoB, re-checking on allergies. It was all very frenetic, as though they only had a fixed amount of time and were rushing to get everything done. I tried to erase that thought before it had even finished formulating in my mind. My preference was for them to take their time.

Then he appeared... The Anaesthetist... and it dawned on me; that would be a great name for a Gangster. Or at the very least, a henchman. Again, I tried to kick that thought into the long grass. It really wasn't the time for dwelling on gangland *torture for fun* scenarios.

There was still a lot of activity going on around me when an oxygen mask was placed over my mouth and nose. Much more activity than I'd expected. I'd imagined everyone would be ready and waiting and... still, by this point. Perhaps with classical music or an Amazonian rainstorm rumbling in the background. Once the mask had been fitted, it was the familiar routine. I was asked to breathe normally and then count slowly backwards from ten.

Now, as I've mentioned previously if you haven't gone through this before, it's important not to break into a sprint during this phase of play. You don't want to get to one and cause a panic, mostly to yourself, so I was super slow. Previously I'd got to four but, you could never be sure when sleep's soft oblivion would come. Again, I'd wanted my very last conscious thoughts to be of Karina and the boys, so I held an image of them in my mind, even from starting at ten. I recall beginning to feel relaxed, but still very much *with it* at five. At halfway there and still feeling pretty alert, I'd begun to wonder if I'd have to tell The Anaesthetist and risk some sort of retribution. Instead, I held on to the picture of Karina and our boys. They were the reason for me to get myself better and I desperately wanted to be there for them. I got to four and that was my last conscious thought. No drowsiness, no blurring, no fade to black. For the second time in four days, one second I was there, fully present and the next, I wasn't.

I was beginning to make a habit of this.

# 19

# Cyborg

*"And once the storm is over, you won't remember how you made it through, how you managed to survive. You won't even be sure, whether the storm really is over. But one thing is certain. When you come out of the storm, you won't be the same person who walked in. That's what this storm's all about."*

**Haruki Murakami**

It's difficult to say what my absolute first memory was as my body burned off the anaesthetic. I have a whole bunch of recollections of the first couple of days after the operation, but not necessarily a solid grip on the order of some of them.

I had an overwhelming sense of gratitude and relief though, once I was aware I'd survived the operation. Although there had been little doubt about my survival amongst my medical team, for me, despite having more belief than hope, the possibility of not waking up, had always existed. Even if that possibility had only been one or two balls out of a hundred.

Obviously, I hadn't wanted to show this or share this with anyone – there would've been nothing to be gained from doing so. My grain of doubt had been that my body had already so successfully deceived me in the recent past, not to mention some brilliantly experienced medical minds. I'd been asymptomatic and, apart from the blockage, physiologically robust for such a long time in hospital. Only to be discharged and have a cardiac arrest 18 hours later. I knew my body could appear to be one thing (strong), whilst being another (trashed). So, whilst I'd been told I was in far better shape than most people going through the procedure, I had wondered if everything was as it seemed.

Prior to the operation, I'd also had an immense feeling of having been so lucky in surviving the cardiac arrest. Not to mention doing so with all my faculties intact. That level of luck was rare, certainly in my life, so I suppose I'd had a niggle that my luck would run out at some point. The scale of the operation may just have proved too much, and the lights would go out.

But they hadn't, and once I'd managed to process that I'd overcome that first *huge* obstacle, even in my groggy, post-op, broken state, I knew I next had to throw everything at getting better. Not that I was in a position to throw anything, anywhere. Rolling my eyes was a workout.

My first recollections were centred on my environment and the person sharing it with me. At some point, I became aware of someone saying my name. It wasn't a voice I recognised but it was soft and sounded very kind. To the right-hand side of the bed, there was a young nurse in white, with long strawberry blonde hair. She had a kind looking expression and I felt I could trust her. I'm not sure why I'd question whether someone caring for me was trustworthy, but I felt safe. The sense of being in safe hands, coupled with the relief of realising I was through the worst, immediately had the effect of relaxing me, and I went back off to sleep.

I've no idea how long I slept for; it could have been hours or seconds, but I was woken by the same nurse, in the same position, talking in the same way, so it was probably more of a long blink. This time she introduced herself. I'll call her Nat. I tried to respond but couldn't. Speech, at that point, was a skill I was yet to relearn. As was breathing. I had an $O^2$ line under my nose but when I tried to talk, it felt as if I only had an egg cup of air to exhale to try and talk on. That, and my throat felt like it had been rasped out by a cheese grater. And not a little dainty throat sized one, at that.

Recognising the problem, I was asked if I wanted some water, to which I nodded. Nat pressed some button which raised my back up into a slightly more sat-up position and held a beaker with a straw in front of me. I gratefully latched on and sucked. Water – nature's medicine. I was glugging away when the straw was suddenly removed, and I was told I could only have small amounts. She was tough, this one.

My room was about 6m x 6m, completely white with a door to my right-hand side, near the corner. I had machines to the left and right of me and I sensed over my head too, but I couldn't be sure of that. I felt surrounded by tech anyway. Unless Nat was talking to me, the room was quiet except for the whirring and occasional buzzing of these devices. I had no idea what they were doing but appreciated that others did and was grateful they were monitoring them.

I was also aware that I wasn't laying totally flat. Nat had repositioned me slightly but even before, my torso had been slightly raised, as had the section of bed underneath my knees to my feet, so I was in a slight bucket position. I could also feel the mattress slowly moving beneath me. It was a slightly squirmy sensation, which is massively underselling it. It really felt quite pleasant, and all told, I was pretty comfortable. Later, I discovered that the air being moving around in the mattress was designed to minimise the likelihood of pressure sores occurring. Whatever it was, it certainly wasn't unpleasant. I'd have one fitted at home. And in my car.

I was also vaguely aware of a squeezing of my right calf a few times a minute. This, I discovered, was a cuff to help with post-operative circulation, as was a Balloon Pump that had been inserted via an incision in my right leg. I hadn't been told this would be part of the post-op treatment and had thought at the time it was some sort of device that was literally inside of my leg. It was only when doing a bit of research afterwards, that I discovered an Intra-Aortic Balloon Pump (IABP) to give it its full name, enters an artery in the leg via a catheter and follows it round to the aorta in the heart. At the end of the wire, a small balloon inflates and deflates with the rhythm of the heart to help take some pressure off it during the early days following a CABG. So now we both know.

In addition to the cuff on my right leg, there were other sensations, noticeable mostly if I tried to shuffle slightly. A quick audit of my body revealed the sources of these sensations. In addition to the $O^2$ tube under my nose and cuff on my right calf, there was also a cuff on my right arm, for blood pressure. I could also feel something on my neck. In fact, two things and they were plumbed into my neck, not merely stuck onto it. They were two clusters of tubes, with colour coded connectors or ports. They clattered together like something Captain Jack Sparrow had tied into his hair... or the dreadlocks of the Predator. These turned out to be Central Lines that go straight into the jugular vein and allow for large volumes of liquid to be injected or withdrawn, during the procedure.

At some point, I had become a cyborg.

My transformation to borg was confirmed when I looked under the sheets. My gown was down to my waist, and I could see three drain tubes coming out of my abdomen, each syphoning deep red liquid out of my body cavity. There were four wires coming out of my lower chest, which I later learned were stitched to the walls of my heart on the inside and attached to a pacemaker on the outside, should it ever be required. Where these tubes and wires entered through my skin, they were stitched in place so couldn't work themselves loose. All entry points had dressings over the wounds, each with the slightest hint of claret showing through the white gauze. Then there was the large vertical dressing itself. Bang in the middle of my chest. The main event. The Big Zip. Thankfully free of any tubes, so that was a plus, although once again, a hint of scarlet was working its way through the gauze.

My left arm had the cannula which had been used for the anaesthetic, but which was now connected to a drip tube leading to a bag of something, suspended high, somewhere behind my line of sight. (You can see I'm getting the hang of this medical jargon.)

I also had the sensation that each time I moved my left leg, something appeared to slightly tug my appendage to the left. When I say slightly, I mean very firmly, but not very far. This description of a firm, short knob tug, may lead you to suppose that it was, if not a pleasant, then not an unpleasant experience. It wasn't. And it didn't take me long to realise it was a catheter deeply rooted in my bladder and exiting to some bag which I knew would be hanging on the side of the bed. I knew because I'd seen dozens of them whilst waiting on the ward. At that point, I was still too reclined to see under my gown though, so I was spared the image of the actual point of entry.

My left leg appeared to be tube-free, which was a plus. I wasn't sure whether it had earned the bragging rights to being unscathed though, as it appeared to have some sort of sock or bandage wrapped around it, all the way up to the knee. Had they had to harvest after all? The sensation of having all these tubes and wires coming out of me conspired to create the notion of being shackled to the bed. It wasn't easy to move, even slightly and if I'm being honest, I wasn't even that *keen* to move, for fear of pulling something out of place, whether external tubes or wires, or worse still, internal stitches. And of course, because I'm such a wuss, there was also the fear of the pain that would accompany either of those things happening.

On the subject of pain, I'm not a fan. As was touched upon briefly with Mr D just prior to the operation, the thought of the post-op pain terrified me. I just couldn't believe all of that cutting, sawing, and slicing wouldn't result in significant pain. How could it not? Of course, there'd be pain relief, but not for one second did I believe there'd be total pain removal. That was quite impossible to accept and was a serious over-selling of the recovery process, in my mind.

However, I was wrong. As I bounced in and out of consciousness, I felt no pain whatsoever. Not in my chest, my legs, my neck... not anywhere. Mind you, I was so smacked off my tits on morphine, I couldn't feel anything else either. I had no idea if I was weeing. I barely knew if I'd blinked. If I'd shat the bed (I didn't), I'd have been oblivious to it. But, whilst pain was noticeable by its absence, I still feared its arrival. Really badly. Sure, I was ok at that point, but it was on its way. It was like waiting for a tsunami and I was the guy standing on the beach admiring the fish flapping on the suddenly exposed wet sand.

Nat was telling me it was important to keep ahead of the pain, but she was unable to increase my intravenous morphine. Bad times. However, if I wanted, she could give me some measure of oral morphine. This, I very much wanted, so lapped up the syringe of medicine squirted into my mouth. Good times.

Each and every time it was offered, I took it. For *The Pain* was on its way. It was only a matter of when it would arrive, crashing through my body like medieval torture. I couldn't tell you how many times I took a shot in the mouth, but it may have been every four or six hours. To say it dulled the senses is an understatement. My eyeballs felt like they were lubricated with Bostik and my eyelids were controlled by a series of pullies and cables. Individual thoughts were long drawn out HIIT sessions, which, by the time I was finishing one, I couldn't recall why I'd started it. Sleep became my BFF. I'd become a 45 played at 33. And I appreciate that to a great many people younger than me, that analogy will mean absolutely nothing.

Early on, I was bemused by my hands and forearms being so massively wrinkle-free and bloated. I could see my chest and abdomen were round and smooth and felt my neck – it was chunky. Nat caught me doing this and asked if I was OK. I was actually a bit panicky and wanted to say, 'Not really. I came in for a heart bypass, but I think my brain's been transplanted into a fat bastard's body.' But of course, I didn't say that, because, given the amount of morphine I was metabolising and my tiny lung capacity, that sentence would have taken me about three days to get out, so I just said, 'Fff-fat.' She explained that I wasn't, it was just water retention from the saline used during the operation and it would flush out over the next few days. Relieved that I was still the decathlete I always thought I'd been, I drifted back into a pain-free slumber. Sometime later when I was back on the ward, I was telling a nurse this story and was told it wasn't uncommon for patients to put on up to 10kg immediately after the operation, due to water retention. Thank goodness someone had the foresight to shove a tube up my urethra. Not something I'd ordinarily feel grateful about.

I don't recall too much about food or eating during this time, although I know I wasn't up for the usual three-course offering. I do have recollections of bowls of mushy Weetabix being offered to me and accepting four or five spoonfuls before shaking my head like a weaning baby. I'm pretty sure that the fact it was Weetabix had nothing to do with it having been early in the morning. Both time and time of day were redundant concepts during this phase of my life.

If my surroundings felt surreal, some of the encounters which took place in the room were even more surreal. One time, I snapped out of a drug-induced slumber to the sound of the door being opened as loudly as a door can be before it comes off its hinges, followed by a man's voice. Similar to the door, the voice was as loud and threatening as it could be before you'd class it as being *out of control*.

'What the hell is going on? Why are you in this room?'

'I'm looking after my patient. Whatever you think has happened, hasn't. Go away,' Nat replied.

'I've got this room booked out – you're in the wrong place,' the guy persisted, as the conversation rapidly became a tennis match.

'Mr Perry is my patient, and this is his allocated recovery room. I don't know what the confusion is but please take your complaint to the desk.' Backhand return from Nat.

'I want this room cleared and cleaned for my patient – you've got one hour.' It was a decent response, but he'd underestimated Nat's ability to cover ground across the court.

'Excuse me Karl,' she said as she got off her stool and approached the door.

'I couldn't care less what you think has happened. This is my patient and I'm caring for him in this room. I'll be passing this on to your Consultant and if you don't disappear right now, I'm calling security,' and quietly closed the door on the guy who stood staring angrily at her through the door window but had no retort. Nat had delivered the verbal equivalent of a baseline lob leaving him stranded and beaten. Either a lob or a right hook. Whatever it was, he hadn't seen it coming and it was Game, Set and Match to Nat. She came back and sat on the stool next to the bed.

'Sorry about that.' Their exchange had broken through the mist of my morphine hit and so far, was the most exciting thing to happen to me that day. Or night. Certainly, post-operation.

'S'fine,' I managed to exhale.

'No, it isn't. And I'll make sure he gets in some real shit for it.'

I could only smile my gratitude, but I was genuinely grateful Nat was not only a nurse but a warrior-nurse who took no prisoners when it came to caring for her patient. Once again, I felt safe on her watch. Once again, I trusted her ability to look after me. Trust is sometimes so overlooked in some quarters of the medical world. And yet to patients, treatment without trust is just a gamble on the treatment. Having got through the operation and with Nat as my protector, I knew all I had to do was focus on recovery and it would come.

At some point during the first 24 hours after the operation, I received my first Doctor's visit, although it wasn't my *Doctor*, it was the Anaesthetist. I recognised him immediately and felt a little disappointed Mr D wasn't with him. I had absolutely no idea what time this might have been, but Nat wasn't in the room.

He was a little curt in his greeting, as he pulled up a stool and sat on the left-hand side of my bed. I was told the operation had gone well and the valve repair had been a success, so I'd be glad to know there had been no need to act on my decision for a tissue replacement. (I hadn't even thought to ask, by that point.) He still seemed sulky I hadn't chosen his preferred option, but I let it slide. He offered very little eye contact preferring to study the tech surrounding me, along with my notes. But then he closed the folder and gave me his full attention.

'I do have some bad news for you though,' he said.

'Wha's tha,' I managed to exhale.

'We discovered some damage to the heart – probably from the cardiac arrest...'

He expanded on this as he stayed for a few more minutes but I can't recall exactly what he said. The general context though was along the lines of the damage being *extensive* and *severe*.

I was overwhelmingly gutted. This was the worst possible news. Until that point, I'd understood everything had gone well, as, 1) I was conscious so had survived the operation, and 2) no one had told me differently.

But now someone who had been in the operating theatre; had seen, heard, and contributed to all the surgical conversations; someone who had been by my side the whole time was telling me the opposite. A damaged heart would mean a depleted quality of life, the almost inevitable prospect of future heart attacks, and in all likelihood, an early death. I'd hoped for, and thought that having survived the operation, following a period of recovery, I'd be back to a normal, fully active life and this whole phase of my life could be firmly parked in the past tense. Something which I'd eventually not give a second thought to on a day-to-day basis. Something that had once happened to me but would ultimately just become a part of my story.

Immediately after he left, another visitor came straight in and stood to the right-hand side of my bed. This was another face I hadn't seen before, and she introduced herself as Sister Somebody... She came close to the bed and lent into me.

'Are you Ok?' she asked.

Speaking was still a luxury I was building up to, so responding was a series of whispers punctuated with gasps for air.

'Nho... just... had some... bad news...'

She nodded. 'Yes, I know. Do you have any questions or want to talk about anything?'

I had about a million questions and wanted to scream, 'What the fuck's going to happen to me?' but that would have been quite rude and once again, my Mum would've been mightily disappointed in me. That was one reason why we didn't chat at that point. That, and my complete physical and mental inability to have what you'd describe as a fluid and coherent conversation. As such, my answer remained short.

'Yea bu... noh now... gonna... rest now.'

The Sister smiled empathetically and nodded.

'Well let me know if you do,' and with a pat on my arm, left me to my thoughts, which were few, but simple.

Emotionally, I felt broken. I felt broken for me, broken for Karina, and broken for my boys and the rest of my close family. This was the worst of all worlds. Surviving the operation only to hear I was the owner of a damaged heart – and all the unknowns that would bring.

But – and there is a but, because somehow, despite how I felt emotionally, my thoughts were elsewhere. I knew there was nothing I could do about this news, at that point in time. I knew it would be wasted effort to be dwelling on it, at that point in time. And what's more, at that point in time, I somehow had a sense of how best to help myself, which was not to focus on the news and all its unknown outcomes for the future. But to focus everything I had on getting better in the here and now. Or rather the *there* and *then*. And getting better meant getting stronger. In the absolute immediate short term, the only things I could do to improve my strength were to sleep, eat and keep taking fluids on. And with that as my focus, I engaged with the first of those three and did so like an Olympian.

# 20

# The Comeback

*"When everything seems to be against you,
remember that the airplane takes off against the wind, not with it."*
**Henry Ford**

At some point, I was woken to discover my surgeon, flanked by two Doctors, stood in front of me. I don't recall seeing one of them ever again but the guy to Mr D's right became known to me as No.2. I saw him many times throughout the rest of my stay in hospital. As Mr D's right-hand man, No.2 seemed appropriate. I doubt very much that he actually was Mr D's right-hand man in any way other than, on that specific day, he wasn't standing on his left.

There were a few pleasantries and I asked what the time was. I was told it was about 1:30pm. I was quite surprised and replied that the operation had been, 'Quite quick then.' (I'd been expecting it to last about 5-6 hours). Mr D then had to break it to me that, 'Today is Sunday and the operation was yesterday.'

Yes of course it was. Why was I thinking anything other than that? Possibly due to the elephantine doses of morphine I was marinating in.

I was told the operation had gone very well and that all aspects of the procedure were completed as he had hoped, including the valve repair, rather than replacement. I acknowledged all this positive information and then managed to get out that I'd heard the bad news though.

'Bad news? What bad news?' Mr D enquired, with a slightly bemused look.

'Tha ma... hart is... badly dam-gd... from th'... arrest,' I panted.

Mr D's expression went from bemused to stern as he quickly glanced either side – each Doctor responding with a puzzled shake of their heads. Mr D settled his gaze back on me and said,

'I saw absolutely no evidence of that whatsoever. Who told you that?'

'Th'aneeth-tist... s been...'

'Tony?!!'

I replied with a nod although I had no idea of his name. I'd only come across one Anaesthetist during my stay though, and I'd definitely seen him three times.

Even in my depleted state, I could tell Mr D was pissed off. Seriously pissed off. I was told to disregard anything about heart damage and that everything had gone to plan. He then left the room at a fair rate of knots quickly followed by the other two Doctors. My surgeon was clearly intent on removing some body parts and scalpels would not be required.

It's difficult to convey just how uplifting this news was. My immediate plan hadn't changed. It couldn't change. There was so little I could do to influence my recovery, but it felt there was more purpose to it now. An undamaged heart meant a full recovery was now, once again possible and I would be doing everything I could to achieve it. Plan A was back on.

Back to sleep, it was then.

But it does beg the question – what the hell was that visit from the Anaesthetist all about? I thought about this at length over the following days and weeks and eventually concluded there could only be four possibilities:

1. The visit never happened except in my imagination. It'd been nothing more than a surfacing of my greatest fears, projected onto someone who I'd felt had been unnecessarily nazzy with me not long before the operation. This imaginary encounter being fuelled by the Shipmanesque dosage of morphine I was metabolising.

2. The visit happened and he'd lied in telling me my heart was basically shagged. Why? I could come up with no other reason than he got a kick out of upsetting patients. Of course, it would eventually be brought up, but he could always deny that he'd visited or if he had visited, deny that he'd said what I claimed. Again, he'd simply point to the fact I was off my threp'ny bits on drugs, well known to cause hallucinations.

3. The visit happened and there was some degree of truth to what he'd said, but nothing like the level he'd stated. Perhaps Mr D had felt the amount of damage was minor, so would have a negligible impact on achieving a full recovery.

4. The visit happened and he'd told the total truth about the damage to my heart, but Mr D hadn't intended to share that level of distressing information, at that stage. Mr D may have taken the view that, if a full recovery wasn't possible, telling me so soon after the operation, may hinder the degree to which I would have thrown myself into at least maximising what was achievable.

So, which was it? What had really happened?

Looking at option 1: I can completely accept my drug use at that moment in time, was at a lifetime high. I was smashing PBs for use of performance unenhancing substances. And as I later discovered, they did indeed come with the added benefit of hallucinations (more on this to come). But the nature of those later hallucinations was very different to my memory of the Anaesthetist's visit. The tangible nature of that visit had been clear. The conversation had been clear. The message had been clear. I had understood exactly what was being said. There was no sense of being in a dream state.

What's more, there was the brief follow up conversation with the Sister immediately following his visit. Had that been my imagination too? Prior to that very short conversation, I'd never seen her before in my life. And yet, I saw her again, two or three days later, in another part of ICU and I recognised her as being the person who spoke to me after the visit. I hadn't seen her between those two times, which begs the question, if I hadn't honestly seen her following the visit, then where could I have recognised her from?

On this basis, I felt comfortable discounting the theory that it had all been a figment of my drug-fuelled imagination.

I had doubts about the second option too. It's a too high-risk strategy for the guy. Think about it: if you get your kicks out of upsetting patients, the chances are, you'd have done it before. This would leave a track record, if not of complaints from patients, then an awareness of your MO amongst colleagues. A reputation would develop and if that existed, I doubt Mr D would have wanted that kind of player on his team. But then again, even a serial killer has to start with their first victim. Maybe I was just unlucky, and I was his first. The second option remained a possibility.

Options 3 and 4 disturbed me, as it meant I had to consider the possibility, that as a result of the cardiac arrest, my heart was damaged to a greater or lesser degree. But damaged, nonetheless. This, I absolutely didn't want to consider. But it's an almost universal truth that if you ask your mind not to think about a pink elephant, guess what you think about? That said, I was confident it wasn't option 4, as Mr D was emphatic he'd seen no evidence of severe damage. It would be difficult to backtrack from that position, so I couldn't believe he would set himself up, to have to do so.

The jury was hung between options 2 and 3. Option 2 just felt too mean and at total odds with the behaviour expected of someone in the medical profession. Option 3 was a little frightening in that I wanted to be the owner of a fully functioning heart and I suspected that even *slightly damaged* could lead to other issues developing.

Throughout my whole recent hospital and wider cardio experience, I'd never been shy of asking plenty of questions to plenty of people but I'm more than ashamed to say, I never once asked any further questions about the Anaesthetist's visit. I never followed up with Mr D and it's interesting that he never followed up with me about it either. I also never followed up with the Sister, although I never saw her again once I'd left ICU. (I didn't even share the story about the Anaesthetist's visit with my family until many months later.)

This, I know, was because I was afraid. I didn't want to run the chance of having any doubt confirmed. If I asked a direct question, I may get a direct answer – and one that I didn't want to hear. It must be the only time in my life I've chosen to live in ignorance. I concluded that if there were any issues with damage, they'd quickly become apparent during my recovery. It would be slow and my capacity to be active would be limited. I'd find out soon enough whether the wind was at my back, or I had a lifetime of headwind to endure. In the meantime, I'd be throwing everything into Plan A and would wait to see how the evidence of recovery presented itself.

During the operation, my lungs were deflated whilst I was on the heart-lung machine, which caused them to stick together. This is expected. At that early stage in my recovery, they remained still mostly stuck together, hence the greatly reduced capacity. To reverse this, I was encouraged to do physio on my lungs during the short spells of being awake. This involved using the Andean-bong I'd seen so many others on the ward attempting to play. At its most basic, sucking air through the tube caused the balls to rise and in the process, caused the air sacs in the lungs to separate. It seemed a simple enough challenge, but I might as well have been asked to play the Bagpipes.

Getting the balls to the top of the tubes was an impossible task and my early attempts barely caused them to wobble. I'd been told, if left to their own devices, it was likely some parts of my lungs may never fully re-open, which would mean a limited capacity. Which in turn would mean a compromise on the quality of my future life. This option didn't form any part of my Plan A, so I embraced the challenge.

In fairness, *embraced* is way too strong a word. I totally hated having to do it. My lungs burned as they approached the limits of what they could hold. I was asked to try and play this tuneless windpipe twice, about four times an hour whenever I was awake.

Progress was slow. During those early days, the balls took on the properties of blu-tac covered steel ball-bearings. The longer they stayed at the bottom of those pipes, the longer I'd be talking in a whisper. Gradually though, the balls began to defy gravity. Only slightly, but I was elated at first seeing this sign of progress. Progress, in any form, was my primary goal, so anything which provided evidence of this was a massive boost.

I only have the briefest of recollections of Karina's first visit, which was on the Sunday evening. It was only for a few minutes and there was only really a very short exchange of words (Karina) and whispers (me). I was absolutely exhausted - or sedated - but I felt really connected with her. I had no energy to convey it so simply asked that she just touched my face. She cupped her hand, and I lent my face into it. It felt warm and soft but most importantly to me at that time, familiar. I was in a whole new alien place and feeling that familiar warmth and softness was reassuring. Reassuring enough to send me straight back to sleep.

I woke on Monday to find a different face greeting me. It was a nurse in scrubs who introduced herself as let's say, Anita. She explained that Nat was off shift that day, so she would be looking after me. I was gutted. I'd only been fully aware of Nat for less than 24 hours, but I trusted her. I'd seen her in action. She was tough and focussed and kind – and given I could barely function, these were just the qualities I needed.

I needn't have worried though. Anita quickly proved herself to be every bit as tough and focussed and kind as Nat had been. I'd felt pretty crap when I'd woken up. Not in terms of feeling pain. More like a bad hangover. I had a muggy head and my mouth tasted bitter. I mentioned this to Anita, and was told it was probably caused by the oral morphine – did I want to cut back on it?

*Hell no!* I wasn't risking actual pain over a bit of grogginess! That said, how I was feeling, crushed any semblance of appetite so when I was offered my mushed-up Weetabix, I declined.

Anita was having none of it. 'Karl, if you don't eat, your body won't repair itself and when your family visit, you'll look like you've gone backwards. Is that what you really want?'

Oh, she was good. She knew which levers to pull. I absolutely wanted my family to see an improvement in me, on every visit. It's underestimated how much a patient feeds off the tone given by their visitors. I wanted evidence of progress. Sunday night had been a mere cameo appearance by me and I was keen to improve my performance.

In the afternoon, I had a visit from No.2 who was very happy with my progress and set about removing the balloon pump. This I took as a step in the right direction. My first tube being removed was symbolic. A release from one of my many shackles. Tubes added = not good. Tubes taken away = one step closer to normality.

I was told to lie very, very still whilst they removed the line from my leg. This was one of the few things still well within my skill set. In fact, a little earlier, Anita had asked if I was comfortable as I looked tense and rigid, the whole time. All told, I was very comfortable. The slow manipulations of the mattress and near-permanent state of being spanked off my bonce with morphine made for a not too unpleasant experience. But I was also in a near-permanent state of fear of undoing something if I moved in any way. I felt sure a stitch somewhere would pop, or my chest would just come undone if I even relaxed any part of my body. So, my whole body was clenched tight and for a while, I wore my shoulders as earmuffs.

Back to the balloon pump removal. The line came free from my leg via a tiny incision in an artery. As I knew from experience, arteries aren't fans of incisions of any size and No. 2 knew this too. Hence the enormous amount of pressure he applied to the gauze placed over the incision.

After a few minutes, he gently peeled the gauze back to see if the wound had sealed. The arc of claret over the sheets and my gown suggested not. He apologised again and redoubled the pressure. It was about 30 mins before he was finally happy the wound had sealed, and a pressure dressing was applied. I really hadn't been that fussed whilst this was all going on. It was once the procedure was over and I was on my own that I began to feel some anxiety. It dawned on me that this was yet another reason to stay as still as possible; to avoid *unsealing* my latest wound. If that were to happen, I could painlessly leak myself out onto the mattress and be unconscious in minutes, without anyone even knowing.

I was on guard at the door of my own body all the time, just to make sure that, in a moment of relaxation, I didn't roll onto my side and spill my insides out onto the floor. Hence, the permanent state of rigidity.

My goal of achieving a complete lack of movement wasn't matched by my medical team. Anita advised I was due a visit by my Doctors later in the afternoon and they'd really like to see me sat up in a chair. I gave her my best attempt at a sarcastic laugh, but to my complete disbelief, she was totally serious. I genuinely had no idea how this could even be a consideration. I could barely wriggle, I believed. I was devoid of any strength, was shitting myself I'd split open at any moment and was spanked to my eyeballs on crack. Allegedly.

If you've ever wondered how they got Davros into that bottom part of a Dalek, I could explain in graphic detail. The finished result didn't look too dissimilar either. The chair was a wheelchair of sorts but with an elevated seat and supports for my head and shoulders. It was the tubes which added the final Davrovian touches: the seven or eight dreadlocks plumbed into my neck; the three drains carrying their deep red liquid cargo into their respective half-full suction bottles; the catheter which by now was constantly syphoning urine out of my bladder into a bag, very visibly hooked onto to the side of the chair; the sticky-backed electrodes attached to my chest and the wires connected to a heart rate monitor; the drip, intravenously feeding me my pain relief and let's not forget the four wires stitched into my chest which were attached to the external pacemaker, (thankfully still unrequired, by that point). With the balloon pump having been removed, it was only approximately 20 tubes and wires connected to or disappearing into my body.

Couple this with the extreme bloating, and the rolling eyes of someone who could've listed solvent abuse as a hobby, and you probably didn't have me at my best.

Only two visitors were allowed at a time and Karina and George came in first. I can't recall too much apart from Karina being really pleased at seeing me sitting up in a chair. *Sitting up* is probably stretching the definition of the words to their very limits. Propped up and strapped in, would be more accurate.

Ben came in with his Aunty Sarah. Even in my morphine addled state, I could tell as soon as he'd entered the room, this was even more challenging for him than it was for me. My Davrovian make-over was hardly easy on the eye. But then, it couldn't have been easy, at 14, to see your Dad looking like that. I certainly wouldn't have liked it and didn't particularly like, being it.

The following day heralded further milestones indicating progress. I was told that as things were going so well, I was to be moved out to a different part of the ICU. So, still within the same department, but into a room with six or seven other patients. A sort of, Slightly Less Intensive, Intensive Care Unit. This was the best news I'd had since waking up. But prior to being transferred, the two drains either side of the central one would be removed, as they hadn't gathered any sludge for 24 hours or so. This was also great news. 10% of my tubage being removed in one go.

By this point, Nat was back on shift and both her and Anita set to work on me. The stitches holding the first drain tube were snipped. I was told to take a deep breath and then exhale. Another deep breath in and then they would remove the tube when I next exhaled. No problem. Exhaling was yet another skill well within my locker.

When I exhaled and the tube was pulled sharply backwards and out of my chest cavity, it was as if my lungs were being sucked out through my diaphragm. Upon removal, the tube secreted deep red, gunky liquid onto my body, which was quickly wiped away. The pain, although short-lived and over within a second, was more intense than I'd expected and was a sensation I'd never felt before. It really was a thoroughly unpleasant experience. There was also the knowledge that in just a few seconds, the next one would be pulled out. But just before that happened, there was a little interlude as the stitches on the wound where the first tube had been, were tied up. This only took 30 seconds or so but felt like an age as I anticipated whether the removal of the right drain would be as uncomfortable, more uncomfortable, or possibly, with a good wind, even less uncomfortable as the left one had been.

The second drain removal was a near mirror performance. Intensely painful. There was still one drain stitched into me and I knew, at some point, that too would need to be yanked from my chest cavity. But that was for another day. For now, we were finished. I was so relieved that phase was over and I'd managed to shed two further shackles. It was like completing a challenge to progress to the next level of some twisted Escape Room. Which bizarrely, pretty much describes how I felt about the whole experience during the next phase of my supposedly de-escalated period in Slightly Less Intensive, ICU.

# 21

## DefCon 1

*"Fear doesn't shut you down; it wakes you up."*
**Veronica Roth**

It was early Tuesday afternoon when my bed and I were wheeled out of the room which had been my world for what had felt like weeks but had only been three nights. Karina and Sarah accompanied me, and Nat was there to manage the hand-over.

There were six other patients in my new home, all well-spaced out and surrounded by the usual tech. At the opposite end of the room was the Nurses' Station. This was a positive thing; it meant a quieter life. Less traffic. No 24-hour running commentary. Greatly reduced passive-aggressive sniping about colleagues' rotas. It still went on, but given the distance, it was much quieter.

To the right of the Nurses' Station, there were double doors to another ward: *Even More Slightly Less Intensive, ICU.* They probably had a snappier name for it, but that became my next goal. Getting through those doors. That's what I had to focus on. That, for me, would be further proof of progress.

I'd been told my care was being handed over to Nurse G – let's call him Gerry. He had a tough act to follow and I was disappointed to be leaving Nat and Anita. They'd both been everything someone in my position had needed: super-caring and attentive; encouraging;

they'd stretched my expectations of what I could, or rather should, be achieving. They certainly took no shit, from me or anyone else and of course, they'd dispatched their clinical duties to the highest of standards.

You might assume these qualities could and should be attributed to all nurses or indeed, all clinical staff. As my hospital stay went on, I began to realise this was not the case. There were wide variations in how clinical staff delivered their roles and as most of my day-to-day contact would be with nurses, it was amongst them where I experienced the greatest variations in approach and style.

I called it *Nursecraft*.

For me, nursecraft wasn't necessarily just about the *what*; the ability to find a vein, take blood pressure, issue medication or the million other clinical and care-related tasks nurses engage in daily. Although having the skills to carry out required tasks does contribute to nursecraft, for me, it was primarily about the *how*. How those tasks were carried out; how nurses fulfil their roles; how they interact with patients, visitors, and other staff.

There are approximately 1.3 million employees in the NHS which makes it the largest employer in Europe and one of the largest employers in the World. There is a commonly held belief, often promoted across social media, that *everyone* who works in the NHS is utterly exceptional at their job. Spoiler Alert! Imagine a graph where you apply a normal distribution curve to the 1.3 million employees, with some sort of generalist performance measure such as *delivery excellence* or *patient experience* along the bottom axis and employee numbers on the upright axis. It's very apparent, this clearly can't be the case.

1.3 million is a pretty big sample size so should be pretty accurate in terms of statistical significance. In very broad, generalist terms, this means the curve tells us there's a smaller proportion of shining beacons to the far right, a small proportion of staff-of-concern to the far left with the majority being the competent average performers in the middle. That's not me making a stand-out statement. That's just statistics folks! The same would apply to teachers, games designers, driving instructors, event organisers, authors...

I know I'm at risk of starting a Twitter pile-on and sounding incredibly ungrateful, given the amazing care I almost always received; not to mention how the NHS had to manage the enormous stresses generated by the Covid-19 pandemic. Without a doubt, the nation (and in this case me) owe the NHS a massive debt of gratitude.

I also appreciate that staffing and funding can have a big impact on the level of care patients receive, but that's not a nursecraft issue. This is about the basics. It's about micro engagements with patients and visitors; tiny actions, words, tones, attitudes, incidences of pro-activity, or not, that can make an exponential difference to patient experience.

The harsh reality is, no organisation of that size can hand on heart, claim all its employees are of an equally high, *exceptional* standard. Amongst 1.3 million employees, there will be a complete cross-section of performance, care, and dedication. Anyone suggesting otherwise just doesn't want to cause offence or can't bear the thought of being singled out for expressing this honest opinion. The people closest to this world; those who work within the NHS, will know this to be true. They will see the full spectrum of what colleagues bring or don't bring to their roles, on an hourly basis. I know because I've asked them. Likewise, any patient who's spent a reasonable length of time in hospital is under no illusion that everyone in the NHS is an elite operator.

Just to be clear, I'm not targeting nurses here. Nursecraft is applicable across the whole spectrum of roles within the medical and caring profession. My point is that just because people work in the caring industry, it doesn't mean they all care to the same level. Or in some cases, even have the skill set to be there. Read on.

Nat and Anita's nursecraft *was* exceptional. I 100% accept that for them, I was simply one patient of thousands for whom they will have cared for. They won't even remember me and nor should they. But I'll never forget them and what they did for me. I'll be eternally grateful to them; such was their standard of nursecraft.

By the time of my transfer, I was yet to come up with the word *nursecraft* but the concept and its relevance began to take shape over the 24 hours following my move to Slightly Less Intensive, ICU.

There was an air of the theatrical about Gerry. He talked louder than was necessary and punctuated his chat with mock emotion. Let's call him flamboyant.

I couldn't have cared less. I just wanted to be cared for. Besides, being downgraded to Slightly Less Intensive, ICU was a massive win and as sorry as I was to be leaving Nat and Anita, this was another giant leap in the right direction. More evidence that my recovery was on track. Progress was being made.

You may assume all staff in ICU would know each other but Nat and Gerry clearly hadn't met. He very loudly introduced himself and Nat, task focussed as ever, quickly moved on to brief him on my history and medication, just a few metres from the bed. Gerry peppered the briefing with what he probably regarded as *funnies*. During this time, Karina, Sarah, and I were talking quietly but his volume would frequently dial-up, turning our conversation into a series of smaller, interrupted conversations. Once the clinical handover was complete, Nat popped over to say goodbye and wished me luck. Gerry stepped in, put his arm around her shoulder, squeezed her upper left arm and gave her a little shake, saying, 'Don't you worry honey – I'll be taking good care of him. He's in safe hands with me.'

Good to know. Nat deftly spun out of the squeeze and headed off, back to ICU Proper.

Now we had Gerry all to ourselves. Joy.

I was due some medication, and I had my six-hourly hit of oral pain relief, which had been keeping me in a very pleasant, near-permanent state of numbness. But around this time, I also began to register a growing sense of paranoia, woven in with the numbness. Perhaps the change in environment and carer had triggered it off. But I doubt the cumulative effect of pain killer meds bathing my brain, helped.

Gerry was chatting away to Karina whilst preparing my meds. A Doctor suddenly called him away to another patient he was also caring for. I wasn't sorry to lose his attention. I don't naturally gravitate towards loud, peacock types at the best of times, but with 18 or so wires and tubes shackling me to the bed, there was no means of escape. If a breather meant him looking after someone else, that worked for me. By then, I was spending more time awake than asleep during the daytime and my drive to recover, meant that, even in my morphed-out state, I'd been paying attention to what meds I was taking. I knew the last batch he'd given me had been missing a small white tablet, a Beta-blocker, as he'd been called away before finishing preparing the meds. I'd mentioned this to Karina whilst Gerry was with the other patient.

Sometime later Gerry returned, and Karina raised it with him. He was very sure it'd been included but checked the log. Imagine his surprise to see that he'd not recorded it as given. He was very apologetic, congratulated us on our vigilance and asked Karina if she had a medical background. (By then, we were referring to Karina as *Nurse Perry*, given the number of times she'd been asked that question.)

This man was my carer. As far as I was concerned, his role was to deliver me to the next level so I could escape the Escape Room. Why then, having been downgraded into Slightly Less Intensive ICU, did I feel the need to increase my vigilance? I raised my alert level to Def-Con 2.

Karina and Sarah left to get something to eat, and I felt I couldn't allow my guard to slip. I kept an eye on Gerry. It made interesting viewing too. A female nurse was walking across the length of the centre of the room towards the Nurses' Station. She walked with the speed and purpose of someone who was already late in getting from A to B but also had visits to C, D & E on her mind. The Gezza dashed over to her saying (loudly, obviously), 'Hey Ems – did you hear about my near Freudian Slip?'

My first thought was, 'Right – so it wasn't even a Freudian Slip, just some shite you were dribbling.' This was good news. I was beginning to reconnect with my ability for picking people up on talking bollocks. I must have been on the mend. Albeit slowly and with increasing levels of paranoia.

Nurse Emma didn't break her stride to the Nurses' Station. She appeared to dispassionately answer in the negative, but with no request for further information on said near-miss slippage of the Freudian variety. Gerry was matching her step for step and took her lack of awareness as a green light to start his anecdote. On a scale of 1 to 10, I'd say Nurse Emma's interest in this anecdote, looked to be somewhere around absolute zero. Absolute Zero can also be expressed as minus 273°C. Which, by coincidence, was also the level of warmth she emitted at having to hear this tale of mirth and faux pas. If the antennae of a guy spanked to his nipples on morphine, two days after regaining consciousness following open-heart surgery can pick this up, I was puzzled as to why Gezza, the man responsible for my care, couldn't.

Emma scribbled away onto forms and paperwork whilst Gerry relayed his hilarious piece of self-publicity. To her immense credit, she gave the occasional response so as not to be outrightly rude but overall, I'd have described the encounter as *arctic*. As Emma made good her escape and Gerry grabbed some *Heroes* from the tub at the end of the Station ('one for now and a few for later'), two things occurred to me: I wondered if Emma's scribbles had just been her trying to get a pen to work but felt that was more rewarding than engaging in Gerry's tale? Secondly, why, despite now being on the other side of a large room to me, had his volume seemingly not decreased?

Whilst he was still at the Nurses' Station attempting to hold court with yet another Jackanory session, a Doctor entered the room and started a discussion with him. It didn't last long but by the time the Doctor left the room, Gerry looked a little deflated. I have an idea what was being discussed but I'd be speculating. That said, I escalated my alert level to DefCon 1.

When Karina and Sarah returned, I gave them a breathy lowdown on recent events, which unsurprisingly, concerned them. More worryingly, within minutes, Karina discovered some unplugged wire on my bed, so asked Gerry if said wire should be connected to something.

'Oooo... yes it should,' and duly re-attached it. He then once again asked Karina, 'You're very good, you – are you sure you don't have a medical background?'

When pulling these memories together, none of us can specifically remember what the wire was, or what it was supposed to be doing, but we all recall the incident. Neither Karina nor Sarah were happy leaving me that evening.

My evening meds were all accurate, but I decided to half my dose of oral painkiller. Partially because I was very aware I'd settled into a near-permanent state of spankdom, but primarily because I felt I needed my wits about me. My world had become a very different place. Admittedly, a significant driver for this sense of needing my wits was my drug-induced paranoia. I felt threatened and anxious. Not the best double act to be managing when getting over heart surgery.

But I'd also witnessed that care provision meant different things to different carers. Nursecraft can be learned, but for some, it's just second nature and is part of their innate ability to do their job to the highest standard. Gerry was very subdued for the rest of his shift which finished at 8 pm. Our paths had only crossed for about six hours of my life but just as with Nat and Anita, I shall never forget him. Only for very different reasons.

I'm aware that I've painted a pretty negative picture of the guy and with hindsight, I feel a bit sorry for him now. There was plenty he got right, but I don't think his personality sat well with the role he was tasked to fill. Or perhaps he created the drama and loudness around him to mask his anxiety of working in a high-pressured environment. It can't be easy to be top of your game, 100% of the working day, in a high-pressure environment such as ICU. But that's kind of my point. Of all the hospital environments, staff in ICU need to be top of their game. Perhaps he was just a round peg in a square hole and would have been better suited to a ward.

I don't recall much of my next nurse. She seemed pleasant enough, but I was pretty much out for the count not long after the handover. I was exhausted. Whatever adrenalin had been generated whilst at DefCon 1, had rapidly drained away and my alert level wound back to somewhere between DefCon 3 and being completely unconscious. That said, that Tuesday night proved to be one of the most bizarre of my entire life.

# 22

## Escape Room

*"Everything will be okay in the end.*
*If it's not okay, it's not the end."*
**John Lennon**

That Tuesday night I slept well, in the sense I went to sleep very quickly, very early and I suppose very deeply. But then I woke in the early hours of the morning. Whatever time the phrase *middle of the night* refers to, this was it. There was only a faint glow from the Nurses' Station and the myriad of blinking lights from bedside machines, diligently going about their jobs. Noise was mostly absent apart from muted beeps and occasional whispered voices.

My obs were still being taken at regular intervals throughout the night, so it wasn't unusual to feel a blood pressure cuff being placed around my arm, followed by the tightening grip and then hearing the *pppffffffff...* as I slumbered. During one such routine visit, I dozily turned my head to glance at the nurse and froze. My body stiffened and my breathing halted mid-inhalation.

There was no nurse. Where a nurse should have been, stood a shiny human-sized insect. An upright grasshopper of some sort; bright yellow in colour with red markings. Clicking as it released the cuff from my arm.

As casually as I could, I slowly turned my head away, hoping it hadn't realised I'd seen it. Or it's true form at least. As I tilted my head, I could see half of the rest of the room and another four or five of them. Humanoid insects – some with patients, some at the Nurses' Station. I waited until the one by my bed had shuffled off and only then dared to turn my head back for a better look. Including the one that had left me, there were another two. So maybe seven in total. Eight tops. Seven or eight upright, humanoid grasshoppers, watching over a room of incapacitated men.

Shit. This was why I'd been feeling so bad. So spaced out. They'd drugged us and were experimenting on us. These were the only logical conclusions to draw. But why? Were they harvesting organs? Testing drugs? Keeping us as food? The room had an eerie, otherworldly, cold laboratory-like aura to it. There seemed to be a sinister, neon glow pervading all areas of the space. A bit like how a commercial kitchen may look in the dead of night.

I vaguely recalled having had an operation but was beginning to think I'd been *taken* somehow. Or tricked. Maybe they were the ones that had operated on me? They clearly shape-shifted themselves to appear in human form but for some reason, I had the ability to see through their rouse.

Oh no... my grasshopper was coming back with something in its hand. I scrunched my eyes tightly shut and clenched my whole body as I felt it put something in my ear. It must have been a probe. Or some part of its mouthpiece. They wanted my brain. Understandable of course. So did I. The clicking sounds intensified. As I braced for pain, I decided to be brave, and as one last act of defiance, opened my eyes and fixed my stare on it. I wanted them to know, I was on to them, and that we humans will never just roll over and die as cowards.

My eyelids lifted and the room seemed darker. Less neony. Less glowing. More like I remembered it. The nurse, whom I recognised as the one who'd taken over from Gerry said, 'Sorry for waking you, Karl. I'm just taking your temperature,' as she took the thermometer out of my ear. No clicking. Actual talking. And she was very human-looking. It was a good likeness. If I hadn't known better, I might have fallen for it. But I didn't. I muttered something – I was playing along with it; acting dumb, like I was confused. I suppose I was a little confused but also relieved to see a world I recognised, even if I knew it to be fake. A cleverly crafted illusion, designed to mask their evil deeds.

I was annoyed with myself for feeling relief in the presence of this shape-shifting shyster when I knew it to be a sham. I closed my eyes again to berate myself when WHAM! I was straight back into the neon glowing, other-worldly, experimental room staffed by human-sized, bi-pedal grasshoppers.

WTF?

I opened my eyes again.

Darkened room and nurses.

I closed them.

Back to the land of the neon glow and upright, supersized tarantula food.

Clever. Very clever. But I'd worked it out. So, they only put the front on when we open our eyes. When we close them, that's when they drop their guard, and we see the real deal. I found this to be the case even when I blinked. Which was disturbing, to say the least.

I say *we*. I assumed the other guys in the room had surely noticed what was going on but were also pretending to be asleep. Buying time. Sensible.

Being the youngest of the other patients by a country mile, I was probably the fittest. No doubt they'd be looking to me to get them out of there. I'd need to get a message to them – to let them know, that I knew. I'd start with my immediate neighbour. I just needed to get his attention somehow. I was going to alert him by throwing the rubber dog toy that had suddenly appeared in my hand... but just as quickly, it disappeared.

My thoughts then turned to the escape plan. How to get out of there, without attracting attention. I was convinced there was a window immediately behind me and the room was on the ground floor. What's more, I was pretty sure this whole space was inside our local Town Hall. All I had to do was jump through the window and I'd know which road I was on. From there, I could run home to where everything would be normal. Or just to be on the safe side, I'd head to the house we last lived in, in 2003, 17 years earlier. That'd throw them off the scent. Then I'd alert the authorities. Or pest control services.

Before I could leap through the glass window though, I'd have to pull all the tubes and wires out of my body. There was probably an order to do it in. But I wasn't stupid. The drain and the catheter drilled into my bladder would have to come with me.

This dead of night strategising was beginning to take its toll, so I decided a quick nap was in order, to get my strength up. I'd break out in the morning when they were changing shifts. Good idea. I'd catch them off guard. I should be home for lunch.

I was hangover-tired when I next came to. It was morning and my nurse was once again taking my obs. She was most definitely in human form and gave no hint of preferring to click than talk. Perhaps it'd all been a dream. But perhaps not, so I elected not to share my dead of night insight. Just in case. I wasn't going to give away my home advantage.

But I also made the decision there and then, to discontinue the top up pain relief and just see how I got on with Co-codamol – and only if I needed it.

The giant, bipedal grasshoppers have never shown themselves since, but to this day, I remain vigilant.

And I've developed an aversion to neon.

# 23

## Any Win's A Win

*"Enjoy the little things, for one day you may look back
and realize they were the big things."*
**Robert Brault**

The morning I decided to give up drugs, well *a* drug - the grasshopper inducing one, proved to be a busy and eventful one. By the end of it, I was pleased I hadn't carried through with my overnight plans to break for the border.

Although I was weary from my dead of night adventure, for the first time since the operation, I woke up hungry. You don't have to attend medical school for seven years to recognise this as a good sign. My body needed fuel because it was burning up energy healing itself. There wouldn't be a Savoy grilled breakfast on offer, but it really didn't matter. Just looking forward to feeling full again, was a bit of a novelty for me.

I had a bowl of Weetabix, toast, orange juice and a mug of tea. Just a basic breakfast but the anticipation of it, eating it and feeling full after it, rounded on me as though it was one of the best meals I'd ever had. Recognising this shift in my body's needs and knowing I was doing whatever limited things I could, to help myself get better, lifted me immeasurably. Outside of realising I hadn't been experimented on by human-sized, upright grasshoppers, this was the first win of the day. The first of many.

My overnight nurse had gone by 9am and another new face introduced herself. She was a little gruffer in her tone, not one for small talk. *Task focussed* shall we say? That was fine with me. I just wanted to be cared for. So probably not as high on the nursecraft stakes as my overnight nurse (despite her shape-shifting thing), but compared to Gezza, she was a giant of medicine. All was good. And there was the offer of a wash.

By then it was Wednesday morning and my operation had been on Saturday morning; four days prior. I had the vaguest of recollections of being given a wash in ICU Proper, but couldn't recall who by, or when. Just that various bits of my body were made wet with warm water, wiped, and dried. So, I guess I wasn't entirely Stinky Pete, but it'd be good to freshen up.

I wasn't sure how much I'd be able to do but it turned out my new nurse would be the one doing the washing. This is the closest thing you can get to a Spa treatment, when in ICU, so it's not to be sniffed at. She even did my neck and face, working around the Pirates of the Caribbean dreadlocks hanging out of my neck. But then in her gruffest tone, she said something about *privates* which I didn't quite pick up.

'Sorry?'

'You clean your *own* privates,' delivered at a volume Gerry would've been proud of. It was the tone accompanying the volume, though, that concerned me most. A tone which, anyone nearby, could easily have misinterpreted as her disgustingly responding to a request, by me, for her to wash my privates. I also felt the emphasis on *own* unnecessarily added to this potential, misinterpretation. Her nursecraft score was in freefall.

Fortunately, no one rushed towards me with the offender's register and a pen. I responded that naturally, I'd attend to my own privates; but I asked that she gave me some privacy to do so. (This dignity thing works both ways, nursie.) The curtain was pulled around my bed and the bowl and wipes were left on the table next to me.

I hadn't really had an inspection of the kit down there since the op. In my cracked-out state, I'd occasionally glanced when moving the catheter slightly, but not taken a full inventory. I'm not sure what I was expecting but what I wasn't expecting was a shiny dome of swollen black, blue, and purple. In nothing other than location did it resemble the scrotum I'd come to know and love over the years. Once again, my poor nut bag had, for some reason, been mistaken as a punch bag. I have no idea why. Maybe someone's job was also their hobby. There was also dried blood where the catheter entered my body. This I could rationalise a little more. That's assuming it was *my* blood. Given the scale of everything else that had been done to me and bearing in mind this was not the first time I'd woken to discover I'd been genitally mutilated, I shrugged it off.

So, despite not recognising my own genitalia, I felt so much fresher after the wash. It's amazing how much better you can feel, just by being full and clean. The second win of the day.

Shortly after the wash, my old friend the Davros wheelchair arrived. I wondered if we were going for a spin somewhere exciting but alas not. A couple of more mature female physios had brought it as they wanted to assess my capability of moving from the bed to the chair. They gave me some assistance admittedly, but it was largely just reassurance, which was a pleasant surprise. I could mostly transfer myself, albeit very gingerly. They loaded up the catheter bag, drain and mobile pacer onto the wheelchair, removed the ECG leads and O$^2$ tube from under my nose and wheeled me to the middle of the room.

'Right – showtime. Let's have a walk to the Nurses' Station,' said one of the physios, with the casualness of asking a stranger if they had the time.

'Walk?' I replied as though I was being asked to set off on a 10K. Or eat my own shit. Or perhaps both. 'But I haven't walked yet.' As soon as the words had left my lips, I knew they sounded pathetic, which was exactly the look the physios gave me. These two were old school, I could tell.

'By the time we've finished with you, you'll be breakdancing.' There it was – the old school bants. They got me to my feet and were holding all my tubes and wires to one side, whilst my nurse pulled my gown around me and tightened it up so as not to reveal any low hanging (now purple) fruit.

'Take your time, just find your feet. Let the blood move around your leg muscles for a minute. If you feel a bit dizzy just sit back down in the chair.'

I shuffled my weight from foot to foot. It felt fine. No dizziness. So far, so good. 'Where's the walking frame?' I asked.

'Walking frame?!! A young fit bloke like you?! Don't embarrass yourself.'

Just to be clear, in no way would I attribute this directness to poor nursecraft (not that they were nurses – but the term still applies). This is the universally accepted tone and delivery from anyone below the level of Junior Doctor, to encourage patients to push themselves or take on more responsibility. Admittedly, some staff can deliver it better than others, but I was happy with these two. So far.

'I just thought everyone started with a frame. Everyone seemed to start with one when I was on the wards.'

'That's because they were about 30 years older than you. Come on. Stop stalling.'

With a gentle shake of my head, I set off on my first post-op, voyage of discovery. The voyage came with a running commentary as part of the package.

'Don't look at your feet. Stand up straight. Straighter. Don't stoop. Ok, that's good but that's a shuffle, not a step. Can you lift your feet up? Lift them! That's it. And again. And again. No – keep looking forward. You're not going to fall – we've got you. You're stooping. You're never gonna pull at Rockafellas shuffling like that, are ya?' and so on.

It was about 10 metres from the wheelchair to the desk and I made it. I was elated. I was about 8 or 9 years old when I got my 10m swimming badge. Now, 40+ years later, I wanted one for walking the same distance.

It was a weird sensation in that the walking itself wasn't painful at all, but the apprehension and expectation that it would be were overriding my motor skills. After going through the physical trauma of open-heart surgery, I think my body retreated into itself. Or more likely, my mind deliberately restricted what my body did, to protect it from further trauma or damaging the recovery process. If that sounds a bit flighty, all I can tell you is once again, I was afraid of making any movements that would stretch stitches and pop internal or external wounds. Movements like, standing upright, lifting my feet, and taking a step, and another, and another...

The physios gave me the plaudits which I naturally lapped up, followed by, 'Now... let's walk back to the chair, but in the style of a 50-year-old.'

'Oh, fuck right off...' my eyes seemed to say. But of course, they were right. There's no way my chest would rip open and my body unravel its contents onto the floor, simply by standing up straight and walking. If it did, the surgeon's work wasn't fit for purpose and I for one, wouldn't be clearing it up.

So, I turned to face the wheelchair, stood upright, and walked towards it. Not giant strides, but not fairy steps either. And not a shuffle was seen. My thinking was the quicker I did it, the less time they'd have to give me any shit. It worked. This time the commentary was more like

'Whoa...PB coming up, might be a record! Is Norris McWhirter in the house?' (I did say they were old school). I made it to the chair and sat down. They were very pleased, as was I, judging by my smile which was on full beam. I was a bit breathy but managed to get out, 'You never lose it.'

This sealed my third win of the day, and it was only 10:30am. If nothing else happened that day, it would still have been the best day I'd had in quite a while. I was told they'd see me again in a few days and disappeared off to beast some other victim.

The nurse said I should stay in the chair a while to catch my breath, which was good as I was a tad on the jaded side after almost 20 metres of walking. I should have got sponsorship. Whilst the nurse was changing the bedsheets a Doctor visited me; asked all the usual *how are you feeling* questions, read through the notes, reviewed my obs, was delighted to hear I'd just walked and said, 'Right, everything is going very well. I think it's time to move you on.'

What? That was amazing news! Completely out of the blue, amazing news! I hadn't even been in Slightly Less Intensive, ICU for 24 hours and I was being moved through to Even More Slightly Less Intensive, ICU. Outstanding. It was like being upgraded. Or headhunted. Or being called up for Team GB. I had so much to share with Karina! Win number 4!

'There's not far to go,' I said, nodding at the double doors through to EMSLI, ICU.

'Oh, I think we can skip that,' he said. 'You can go straight back to a ward. But before you do, we'll need to take one of those lines out,' pointing at my intravenous neck jewellery.

Wins 5 and 6 in rapid succession! The buzz was amazing. At a time when I wanted or rather, needed proof I was going to be OK, it was pouring in! Rock bottom was beginning to appear smaller and smaller in my rear-view mirror.

The Doctor had an air of authority about him, so I assumed he'd arrange for someone else to remove the line. But no. He did it there and then with me in the chair. I had flashbacks to the dyno-rod drain removal experience, but this was all very painless. I was down to just the one set of neck trinkets. I was shedding shackles for fun. And to think, less than 12 hours before, I was undergoing human vivisection at the mandibles of oversized grasshoppers. Once again, I patted myself on the back for not going through with my escape plan. I'd have missed all the great things that had happened that morning.

The excitement of the morning was catching up with me though, so I was helped back onto my bed for a pressing appointment with the inside of my eyelids. I was allowed to wake in my own time at which point, a young male nurse arrived with a much less Davrovian-looking wheelchair than I'd been acquainted with of late. Although, it was still predominantly blue and covered in the wipe clean material I'd become so familiar with. Even now, seeing those chairs has an effect on me. I can't say they give me the shivers, or I'm buried in flashbacks, but they do stir up memories. Mostly ones linked to worries, uncertainty, and doubt. And the loss of control.

But on this occasion, the memory would be a positive one as it was my chariot out of ICU-land. There's a world of difference between *being in hospital* and *being in ICU*. Perceptually. Physically. Actually. I don't think there can be a more significant change in a patient's status, than moving out of ICU and onto a ward. There's no greater signal to suggest optimism, progress, improvement, increased stability, less risk, a more favourable outcome altogether. There are no absolutes with health or recovery. No guarantees that the direction of travel will only ever be one way. But the de-escalation from *intensive* to just *care* provides immeasurable relief to the patient and those around them. I could feel it myself.

I'd had an unbelievably positive morning. The best I'd had since being admitted. In fact, given the context of being in the post-op phase, probably the most positive morning I'd ever had during my whole cardiac journey to that point. My glass was overflowing with the good stuff. Yet to my complete surprise, I suddenly felt very emotional.

The relief at being downgraded in severity was immense. Overwhelming even. It had never occurred to me that I may have been holding feelings back or had been trying to hide anxiety. But how I suddenly felt at that point in time, suggested something close to that, had been going on, albeit subconsciously. It must have been an autopilot thing. My neolithic brain had been locked in fight mode; protecting me from my own thoughts and emotions, which left to their own devices, could have hampered my survival. My pre-historic technology had been tasked with dealing with a very real 21st-century issue. Either that or my recent considerable drug use had diverted such feelings into an emotional SPAM folder. Whatever it was, I was consumed with relief and gratitude for everyone who had helped me. Even Gerry.

I was in the chair, with all my tubes, drain, catheter bag and pacemaker loaded. My very few belongings, including my mute Andean windpipe, were in a small bag on my lap and I was wheeled towards the exit next to the Nurses' Station. I really wanted to express my thanks to the nurses there. The truth is, I didn't really have any bond or connection with any of them. None of them at that time had been *my* nurse. Nat and Anita were in ICU Proper – a separate area, so it wasn't as if I'd have been thanking them. But the nurses who just happened to be at the Nurses' Station as I was leaving, felt symbolic of all the staff who'd got me that far and I was deeply, deeply grateful to every one of them.

I felt shrunken. I probably looked shrunken. I was on the verge of tears and all I could muster was a raspy, 'Thanks for all your help.' A pathetic gesture against a debt of gratitude that was owed. I'm usually not short of things to say, whatever the occasion, even on the hoof. But I found myself bereft of words. Completely unable to express myself. I think it's the humblest I've ever felt in my entire life.

So, despite a morning of win after win, it was against this emotional backdrop that I was wheeled into my new ward, slumped in a chair, looking more broken and weary than I'd felt in ages. The Nurses' Station was mid-way along the corridor and as we passed it, a face I recognised suddenly exclaimed, 'Karl!!' It was the Sister from my previous visit. I could tell she hadn't said my name as a means of greeting. It sounded more like shock, probably that I was back, having gone through what I had and the way I looked. I managed to move my mouth into something close to a smile but only for a second. I couldn't give any other acknowledgement.

I was wheeled to the end of the Nurses' Station and was immediately spun left, through a door into a room. Unbelievably, a room just for me! It was a decent size, had a large window - not necessarily the view to go with it - but at least there was plenty of light and ventilation, a basin, a storage unit and of course the ubiquitous wipe-clean, high-backed, patient chair. But it was my room. Even in my subdued state, I knew this was another result. Win number seven for the day.

The nurse who'd pushed me round was only a young lad, maybe 21 or 22 years old. I'd seen him a few times in Slightly Less Intensive,

ICU but our paths hadn't crossed to talk. Whilst wheeling me round, he'd been passing the time asking about my family, if I had kids, what they were up to... all the usual, polite, small talk stuff. I'd imagine he'd have done that anyway, but it would have been obvious to him that this patient needed a bit of distraction. We'd struck some common ground over rugby. He still played and our lads play so there was a bit of chat about positions and clubs. I must have been hard work. Once we were in the room, he moved me to the patient chair and was getting me set up, part of which was putting a new set of compression socks on my feet. He was telling me I'd made brilliant progress to be back on the ward, in that way nurses do; always *bigging up* their patients, and I said, 'Yea and getting my own room is a small win.'

Without breaking from his task, he replied, 'Any win's a win and we take them all.'

Everything seemed to stop for me in that second. It was as if I'd just taken an uppercut.

'Sorry, what?'

He stopped faffing with the sock and looked up at me and said again, 'Any win's a win... and we take them *all*,' with a real emphasis on *all*.

'Yea,' I replied absently. But I was reeling. I felt stunned as a realisation took hold.

It'd taken this young lad to give me a sense of clarity greater than anything I'd felt in my entire life. Of course, any win's a win and we *absolutely have to take them all*. A week ago to the day, I was dead.

Dead.

Gone. No longer on the planet or in the game.

The Earth is just a lump of rock in a random solar system, locked in an outer arm of the Milky Way. It's been that way for billions of years, but for some reason, life exists on it and we humans get a few decades of that life if we're lucky. A period that really, is barely a grain of sand in the whole cosmic scale of time. So, for all the billions of years the Earth has been around, billions of people have come and gone. And just like those billions of people who have laughed and loved and cried and lived on the planet before me, my tiny grain of sand had fallen through the timer.

But only briefly. Because for some reason, on that occasion, I was one of the 8% and my grain had bounced back up.

*Any win's a win - and we take them all.*

It was a simple statement. Under normal circumstances, it would've been a truism anyway; easy to accept. But for me – for my circumstances, it felt profound. It felt like I'd been presented with a mission statement. Like being shown the way life should be lived. Big wins are nice. Everyone likes the big wins. But taking *them all* means celebrating the small wins too. And not just the small wins but any win. Every win. What else can life be about? Celebrate anything good, anything positive.

Prior to that moment, I hadn't overly thought too much about the return ticket I'd travelled on regarding my cardiac arrest. Thinking about it had seemed irrelevant and a waste of energy before the operation. The only things I'd needed to focus on were making it to the operation and then surviving it. Then came phase two: recovering from it. The painkillers had restricted my capacity for much in the way of sensible, cognitive activity, so that day, Wednesday, 15th May 2019, was the first time I was able to even think about things with any clarity. And the nurse's comment was the trigger event. Or at least it provided some context to the cardiac arrest, because if the crux of what he'd said was that we should take even the smallest of wins and celebrate them, then what the hell should I do with a big win like being brought back from a cardiac arrest?

That was the first time since the arrest on $8^{th}$ May that I truly, honestly realised; I'd been given the chance of a second life.

# 24

## A Winning Streak

*"Start where you are. Use what you have. Do what you can."*
**Arthur Ashe**

*A second life* wasn't a phrase I'd ever contemplated.

Until that morning, I hadn't been in any state to truly consider my circumstances. Only the night before, I'd been unable to distinguish between a nurse and a genetically modified grasshopper. The downgrading of my severity status - indicated by being back on a ward - was the first real chance I'd had for the seed of this notion to be planted. But once it had, it couldn't be unplanted.

By the time Karina arrived, I was quite emotional, which was at odds with all the great stuff that had happened to me in the previous few hours. I told her about the nurse and *any win's a win* through tears and shortness of breath. (Crying is unbelievably difficult when re-learning to breathe.) I was in a bit of a state for the rest of the day although, it's fair to say that a sense of relief was also feeding into my state of mind.

I was absolutely shattered by the afternoon. Karina had brought clothing and toiletries in and by 5:30pm, she was leaving me in my PJs, eye-mask on and earplugs in, settling down for the night. Sleep arrived at 5:31pm and apart from vaguely sensing one of the nurse visits in the small hours, I slept through until I was woken for break-fast at around 8:30am.

8:30am is unusually late to be woken in hospital but they must have focussed on the bays first. They also probably recognised what I'd needed more than anything, was sleep. I felt pretty good upon waking but then I'd never slept for 15 hours before. Not without the aid of anaesthetic.

Later that morning, a nurse came to empty my catheter bag, which was brim-full of gallons of golden liquid. She told me it was, *pouring out of me*, as she'd already emptied it during the night. This was great news as it meant my kidneys were firing up again. It was true. I'd noticed my hands and arms weren't as bloated and puffy as those first few days following the operation. More evidence. An-other win. One I gladly took.

That first full day on the ward was about re-acquainting myself with the rhythm and routine of ward life. Having my own room meant more space and conversations could be a little more private but the timings of meals, the cleaner arriving, the tea trolley, Doctor visits, were all pretty much the same for everyone. But even going through a full ward day was tiring and Karina ended up leaving me at 6:30pm, in the same state of readiness for sleep as the day be-fore. I was really looking forward to another super-sized sleep, which thankfully, I got.

Over the next few days, the wins arrived thick and fast. My rate of urine output had returned to normal, so the decision was made to remove the catheter. Although I was the last to find that out.

A young French nurse entered my room and closed the door. She already had a blue plastic apron on and was putting on a pair of latex gloves. She told me what she was going to do and asked me to roll the bedsheet back and lower my PJ bottoms.

Jesus. Straight into it. No, *let's get to know each other a bit, first.* One minute I'm working through the 'nines' for the umpteenth time on a sudoku puzzle. 30 seconds later, I'm getting my ol' fella out in front of a stranger.

It all felt a bit clinical, which of course, is exactly what it was. It's a weird, uncomfortable place you find yourself when the clinical world collides with your sense of dignity. Dignity seldom wins. The result for the patient is some form of embarrassment, but with the emphasis on social awkwardness than a sense of shame. She was just doing her job and had probably handled a range of male genitalia in her time. Certainly during her hours of employment, anyway.

She deflated the balloon and with one hand holding my appendage, began to pull the tubing out. I can't say it was painful as such, but the friction wasn't particularly comfortable. But suddenly, as the tube was nearing the end, I had an overwhelming sensation I was going to wee and told her so. More of an outburst than a telling. For a second, I had an awful vision of pissing all over her, the bedsheets and myself, but she didn't even flinch. Not a flicker. Mainly because I didn't, and she'd probably done this so many times, she knew I wouldn't. It was an expected sensation to experience.

Thankfully it was all over very quickly, and this particular assault on my dignity was much shorter-lived than my episode with the vein scanner, which, to this day, if I think about it, still gives me cause to dip my head, cover my eyes, and want to disappear under a rock.

Another very simple but landmark event was the dressing being removed from my chest. Nurses and Doctors had lifted it daily to check on the wound and had all made positive noises, but it had remained covered for the whole time. For me, this was the big reveal. Whatever was underneath would be my permanent visual reminder of what had happened to me. The scar would become my lifelong buddy. An integral part of my story.

I was totally blown away. I'd seen other guys on this, and previous wards and their scars had seemed neat so I'm not sure what I'd been expecting. People who've had open-heart surgery sometimes refer to themselves as being a member of *The Zipper Club*, on account of the scar. But was I really expecting a zip?

Removing the gauze dressing revealed a pencil-thin wound that started well below the second button of a shirt and ran down the centre of my chest to just below what I'd laughably call my pecs. Probably only six inches in total. (So actually, absolutely massive, ladies.) There was some slight swelling around the edges and a little scabbing here and there but astonishingly, very little to suggest what had gone on underneath. I'd expected more stitches too (hence the zip effect) but even they seemed well spaced. I imagined eventually, it would hardly be visible at all. It was a great feeling knowing I wouldn't be slapped in the face with a reminder, every time I looked in the mirror. Apparently, surgery had moved on since the Battle of Trafalgar and I tipped my non-existent hat to Mr D and his team.

Another win was having the final central line removed from my neck. Again, a completely painless experience. I just laid on the bed as a Hungarian nurse removed the line and applied pressure on the wound for around 15 minutes until the bleeding stopped. The remaining cannula in my arm was also removed. This meant that, apart from occasional blood samples taken, the only wire and tubage exiting my body was the single drain stitched into my chest; the four pacing wires (also stitched into my chest), and the wires attached to adhesive pads on my torso, which were connected to the mobile heart rate monitor. It still took a bit of planning when moving from seat to bed and vice versa but I was developing systems and processes. You just do.

Having no catheter meant I could re-engage with the porcelain. Unless it was first thing in the morning and I was still in my PJs,

I'd reverted to wearing my trusty blue lightweight cargo shorts that had served me so well during previous hospital stretches. I must have worn them every day. And with good reason. They were perfectly suited to my needs. The large pockets on the side of the legs could carry all three items either still plumbed into or stuck onto me. The toilet wasn't a great distance – pretty much across from the Nurses' Station, so it was very manageable. Even so, for my first visit, a nurse insisted on escorting me, then stood outside, asking if I was OK.

It's understandable but being asked if you're OK whilst using the toilet, is a bit of a marker that your life ain't what it used to be. On the other hand, not having to use a carafe from your bed or no longer having a tube dangling from your urethra, could only be chalked up as a win.

By the Friday morning though, I was being asked if I'd had any bowel movements. I hadn't really given it much thought, but on reflection, there had been a state of gridlock since the operation, and that had been on the Saturday before. In fact, it was probably the day before the operation I'd last sat down on a toilet. A whole week prior. A full seven days.

OK, so I hadn't eaten much during the early recovery days, but I'd been ramping it up since the Wednesday and I hadn't even felt so much as an urge to take a tabloid to the toilet.

This planted a seed of anxiety in my mind. Not that I thought there was something wrong with my bowels. No. My concern was that when I finally did back one out, it would be akin to passing a breeze block and I'd rip myself clean open. The medical team were looking for confirmation the bomb doors were functioning fine, and payload delivery was being resumed. Every medical person entering the room tagged that enquiry onto whatever else they'd come in for. Which was hourly.

With that in mind and given I was now able to walk to the toilet, laxatives were given to *loosen me up*. Medical teams love to hear that a patient's bowels are moving, which is understandable. It's a robust indicator that the body is getting its nutrients. It's also in no one's interest to have a backlog of loggage. But equally, they don't want the patient to mistime their evacuation, resulting in a Code Brown and yet another job that could have been avoided. Hence, I was told to give myself plenty of time.

By Saturday morning I was beginning to feel somewhat backed up. Uncomfortably so. I decided to shuffle along the ward a few times to see if walking would help move things along. This appeared to have the desired effect, so I shuffled back to the toilets outside my room. To my horror, both were occupied so I hovered a while, but it appeared the occupants were into extra time and the final whistle was still some way off. For me, it felt for all the world like I was heading into injury time. I shuffled a little further along the ward to another set of toilets. I was in luck. One was free, although only recently so. Perhaps only by nanoseconds, as I slipped in and tried to suppress my natural gag reflex in taking in the acrid, poisonous stench I can now only ever associate with an octogenarian, male shit.

Ordinarily, like you, I would have perceived this as an unwelcome environment in which to carry out one's business. Unpleasant yes. But highly motivating. Any resistance was overcome by the need to evacuate ground zero before my skin began to blister and gums started bleeding. An F1 pitcrew would have raised an admiring eyebrow at my turnaround.

Upon exiting the toilet, an elderly chap who appeared to have been hovering some metres away began to approach the vacant WC. I felt the need to warn him, 'That wasn't me - it was the bloke before who did the real damage.' I very much doubt my warning had any suppressive effect on his own gag reflex. I, however, almost glided back to my room, significantly lighter and significantly happier with yet another win.

Especially since it'd been an away win, well away from the area outside my own room.

The Doctors' daily visit began to develop a sense of familiarity, and thankfully so. Usually, there were two or three Doctors. Quite often No.2 and a man I referred to only as *The Greek* plus occasionally another, usually much more junior Doctor. I know *The Greek* was Greek because he told me so during our first meeting. He hadn't been happy about some blood tests not being back and he'd got quite heated about it. He apologised and explained because he was Greek, he wanted everything yesterday, so finds it frustrating when yesterday becomes next week.

I liked him, but I can imagine he wasn't everyone's favourite Pick n Mix. But the familiarity was compounded by the visits becoming thankfully, very uneventful. There wasn't a great deal to report apart from gradual progress. My resting heart rate was still a little high at that stage. It was in the 80s but was coming down daily. Normally it would've been in the high 50s for me, but it was still settling down from being handled and sliced during the operation, so the Docs were happy with the direction of travel. Their focus was beginning to switch to activity and wanting me to try longer walks, beyond the ward corridor and into the much longer hospital corridors. These appeared to have been built by the Romans, so would definitely be a step up. I programmed these marches into my free time, which I was awash with. These uneventful Doctor visits and instructions to *do more* were collectively becoming another win.

There was one visitor, whom I saw every day from Monday to Friday, throughout my whole stay on the ward. He had no medical input to my recovery, but contributed to it, without fail. Some people light up a room when they enter, and some people light it up when they leave. The Rastafarian cleaner was one of the former. He was called Chiko and would breeze in bringing sunshine and a life vibe with him, which just made me smile. I really liked him. I could only understand every fifth word he spoke, but I really liked him. Sometimes he would be singing but even when talking, he sounded like he was singing. He always referred to me as *Mr Karl* and asked how I was. Then he'd embark on his tasks, sharing some aspect of his life – with which he seemed incredibly happy.

One day, he asked what I did for a job. He became very excited when I mentioned event management. He went through his pockets and produced his wallet. After a brief search accompanied by a little excited singing, he presented me with his business card, which suggested Chiko had a variety of commercial strings to his bow:

*Baby Fada AKA Chiko*
*Professional DJ*
*Party, Christenings, Family Days and Funerals*
*Domestic cleaning and special wine also available*

Not just a bringer of sunshine – clearly a man of many talents, although I don't think he necessarily needed to tap under the word *Funerals* saying, 'Veeeery popular.' Did he have insight into my prognosis that was yet to be conveyed?

I was tempted to ask about the *special wine*, but he probably would've produced a bottle from his trolley. Before his next visit, I googled him and found one of his sets on a YouTube channel. When I told him I'd looked him up, he was made up. My room became the shiniest pin on the ward. Not that it was about that. For me, the human connection was welcome, and he seemed genuinely touched that someone had gone beyond saying, 'Hello.' Some people are just in the right job, just at the exact time you need them to be in that job. I still have his business card and I still smile every time I see it.

Mostly though, as I've established, life on a hospital ward means a lot of time for thinking and you have to be careful here because this can go either way. Thinking can quickly transform into worrying. If you're not getting the feedback and evidence you want (even though you may not be getting evidence to the contrary, either), uncertainty settles in. Uncertainty is often the foundation stone for worry. For me though, as the days rolled on, optimism was beginning to settle. I was allowing a thought to take hold. A thought I was beginning to like. I'd begun to allow myself to believe that I really *did* have the chance of a second life.

Now, just to be clear here, I hadn't thus far, lived a life of regret. Neither had I created a prison from which I'd wanted to walk away. I didn't see myself leaving my whole life behind and heading to Tibet to find myself. Equally, I didn't have a hedonistic urge to live every day as a Freddie Mercury birthday bash.

But I was becoming increasingly aware that I'd been presented with an opportunity. It's a cliché granted, depicted in films and books: often people who experience a life event of such magnitude, find themselves with a revised outlook on life. With doors and often opportunities opening up to them which wouldn't have been thought possible, prior to the event.

This was an exciting prospect to me. There was obviously already a major aspect of my life which I'd wanted to change, namely ownership of my event business. So, given I'd felt I was *already* open to significant change, I wondered what any further change would be, and where it would come from.

I resolved to keep my mind open and to try and be receptive to any opportunities I'd have ordinarily dismissed. I wasn't expecting a bolt of lightning moment, but I sensed there'd be some kind of shift. Maybe a series of catalysts, leading to the notion that life from then on, would be different enough to be able to draw a line between before and after, my cardiac arrest.

I knew I wasn't looking for a major re-write of my life, but I was excited that things would, at some point, be different. I had no inkling about how, what that might look like, when it would be... I just had this overwhelming belief that life surely wouldn't just go back to being the same. Surely there had to be something positive come out of this. For me and my whole family. Change, especially change to the unknown, isn't often embraced. But I was absolutely convinced it was coming. The word I kept using was *opportunity*. And that's what excited me most. What was the opportunity here?

In the meantime, I began to think about some changes I could make, whilst waiting for something other than the bolt of lightning to hit. One of my first thoughts was when I did eventually get back into full-time work, full-time would be three days a week at Assured Events. To free up two days would be wonderful. That would immediately shrink the emotional energy I poured into the business and would allow the space for other opportunities to develop. Another would be to throw myself into fitness. I would become *annoyingly fit* for my age.

I was beginning to feel turbocharged and could see the potential for a second life; a very different life, opening up in front of me. How very exciting.

By the start of the following week, proof of progress and recovery was becoming even more solid. The evidence was mounting up, physically and mentally. I felt a world away from where I'd been only seven days earlier. Inevitably though, progress doesn't travel in straight lines and as I'd increased what I did for myself, I'd noticed considerable restriction of movement in my shoulders. They were locked up. Getting my arms even near to shoulder height generated extreme vocabulary.

Remember my previous mention of how quickly muscle wastes away in hospital? 10% a week is quite a rate and what's left, begins to seize up if it's barely used. Aside from the 18-hour sabbatical I'd had at home, I was approaching five weeks in hospital, and it was visibly taking its toll on my body.

Whilst I hadn't been bed-bound for that whole time, my muscles had suffered. And now my post-operational bloat had completely gone, it was very apparent there was less of me coming out of hiding. I was skinnier, weaker, had frozen shoulders and everyday tasks like a stand-up wash were challenging. It's not surprising really. Aside from the obvious lack of activity, Anita had pointed out I'd been incredibly tense in ICU and I should have tried to relax more. This I clearly didn't do; such was my fear of splitting open and my body just draining away through an imaginary grid in the floor. I was by then, paying the price for overriding her considerable medical training, with my own.

I knew it could be reversed, but only if I did something about it myself. Fortunately, I wasn't short of time, so I put together my own physio programme, which sounds much grander than it was. It started by facing and standing close to the wall. I placed my hands flat against it, shoulders width apart and at shoulder height. I then walked my fingers up the wall until resistance and discomfort wouldn't allow any more height gain. And then walked them down, and then back up again. Simple.

Except each time I did it, I was blowing like a weightlifter and drawing sweat like cheese in a plastic bag. I did this three times and repeated it four times a day. The goal was just to get a little bit higher than the previous session. Sometimes it was just a nudge higher, sometimes it was as much as a finger length higher. After a couple of days, I started doing it one arm at a time as I could stretch further. It took twice as long but fortunately, my diary was flexible. During one particularly strenuous finger-walking exercise, I must have been on the limits of human performance and puffing like a whale, as a nurse at the station just outside the door shouted, 'There must be a hell of a lot of candles on that cake, Karl!' That's the thing about nurses. You can always rely on them to take the piss.

The sensation of stretching sinew and tendons was sometimes vomit-inducing, but it worked. My right shoulder freed up after a few days. The left one improved too but progress was so much slower.

As for the walking, I just kept pushing it, adding multiple lengths to the Roman road outside of my ward. It wasn't just to build up my leg and core muscles, there was also cardiovascular stamina to work on. I was racking up the distances and throwing in the occasional stairwell, for hours on end. I was Forrest Gump. But much, much slower.

There was also an outdoor Quad - a garden space, which was very pleasant. Karina and I would sometimes go there and sit in the sun, chat, have a snack, a cup of tea – basically to get some air and freedom. Obviously, I was still carrying my wiring, drain and mobile HR monitor but the freedom was quite welcome. And of course, sitting outside in the sunshine, how could that be seen as anything other than a win? We had some long and earnest chats there. Mostly they were positive, although my winning streak was about to come to an end and darker clouds were gathering.

# 25

## Bumps In The Road

*"The only way to make sense out of change is to plunge into it,*
*move with it and join the dance."*
**Alan Watts**

Despite all the optimism and positivity around progress being made, it was still very early days. My heart was still settling down after a traumatic ordeal. My blood pressure was fluctuating and whilst I was mostly in a sinus rhythm, I'd occasionally still slip into AF, but then revert. I was told to expect this for up to six weeks before a truer picture of my heart's normalised levels would appear. My heart rate though had been fairly regular and was still gradually coming down as we came to the end of the second week after my cardiac arrest. By then, it wasn't uncommon to be around 75bpm at rest.

At just gone midnight on Wednesday 22$^{nd}$ May, I was woken by a nurse asking if I was OK, which I confirmed I was, although I'd rather have been left asleep. The mobile HR monitor attached to each patient fed through to a large screen at the Nurses' Station and mine had just shot up to between 140-150 and triggered an alarm. Now I was awake, I could feel my heart pounding. At 2½ beats per second under no exertion, I was terrified this was the start of something awful. I couldn't shake the thought that such a high rate would be damaging the grafts and valve repair. The pounding was so hard, I could feel it rocking my body in the bed.

An ECG was carried out and the on-call Cardiologist was alerted. The Specialist didn't attend but reviewed the readout remotely and prescribed a range of meds, which were given immediately. A nurse popped in every hour or so, but my heart rate remained at that level until about 7 am when it suddenly dropped to the 70s. When I say suddenly, I mean like flicking a switch. No gradual wind down, it just clicked back in the space of about 3 seconds. My relief was immense. I just hoped that no damage had been caused, beyond loss of sleep. I'd been awake the whole night worrying and monitoring any and every little sensation I felt in my chest, arms, neck... I'd run my adrenaline supply into the ground. The long and short of it was that I was shattered and fell asleep within minutes of sinus rhythm returning.

But hospital timetables wait for no man, and I was woken at 8:30 for the daily change of bed linen and breakfast. I felt wretched with fatigue. This turn of events was a massive mental blow. Until that point, I'd only seen progress. I'd enjoyed the marginal gains of each small win. Not unreasonably, I'd extrapolated my rate of progress and seen myself as some Olympian Adonis; someone who in the not-too-distant future, would be pushing the bounds of human physical achievement, in some hitherto, undetermined field.

This was a considerable setback. What caused it? Was this how it was going to be from now on? Was there anything that could be done to avoid it happening again? These, and other questions I asked of the Doctors when they visited on their rounds. Naturally, they couldn't say for sure whether there'd be a recurrence, although having had one, they thought it likely there'd be other episodes. But again, it was stressed, it wasn't uncommon for this to happen following bypass surgery.

I was gutted. My confidence was shattered. I wanted to be a total success story – for me, but also for Karina and the boys. I'd wanted to take away their worry and for this to happen, was as if I'd climbed all the ladders, only to land on the longest snake on the board.

Karina could tell my mood had changed as soon as she visited that day. Obviously, she said all the right things, but I could tell she was concerned too. She'd be an awful poker player. So, there I was slumped in the patient chair, looking shattered and fed up, when another visitor stepped into the room. It was lovely Anita from ICU just popping in to see how I was getting on.

Bless her. Anita is one of life's good guys. There was no clinical reason for her to visit. She was just caring enough to want to follow up on an ex-patient, during her break. She too, said all the right things. She told me how brilliant I was doing. That I was looking so well. That I should focus on how far I'd already come. She'd been told about the overnight incident and reiterated these things were just a part of the recovery process. It was just a bump in the road. But the road goes on and I would be fine. Karina was holding, squeezing my left hand. I could barely look at Anita as she was talking. I mostly looked at the floor, occasionally glancing up at her. I could feel my lip wobbling. I swear, if I'd fully looked at her to listen, I'd have just burst into tears.

She was only there for about five minutes, but it meant so much to both of us. Whilst I'd been celebrating all the recent small wins, it hadn't occurred to me how I'd feel about or would deal with, something *not* going my way, because I naively hadn't considered that was even a possibility. It was suddenly very apparent that my confidence was paper-thin. Having said that, I still trusted Anita despite no longer being in her care, and also none of the medical team had escalated their level of concern, so I resolved to try and take my cues from them.

Taking your cues from medics is fine, but you rarely see someone in a clinical role flapping. This means you must learn the art of interpreting behaviours, tones and what *isn't* said. This isn't the blackest and whitest means of information gathering. And then of course, if you're presented with alternative evidence, it pretty much overrides any interpretation you may have previously formulated. Evidence such as, my heart rate going through the roof, which it did again, later that day. Another run of several hours, of what felt like, violent shaking of my recently re-modelled heart. More beta-blockers were given along with other meds and my heart eventually calmed down. If only my imagination had. I was finding this whole reverse in progress, incredibly difficult to handle, in addition to the worry about any damage being caused to my still healing heart. I went to sleep that night feeling very tired but with a weight of worry on my shoulders. Having had two episodes already, I was fully expecting to be woken with yet another run of the rapids.

At about 2am, I was woken by one of the nurses once again asking if I was OK. I felt fine and in those first few seconds of consciousness, carried out a full cardiac self-assessment. Hmmm... I didn't appear to be rocking out. If this was just a courtesy call by the nurse, a could feel a strongly worded letter to my MP coming on.

I was then told my heart rate had been dropping lower and lower and was currently at 30 beats per minute.

WTAF?!!

I was really confused. This was new territory. As heart rate problems go, I'd only ever experienced them on the high side. Right from my very first diagnosis of AF, the issue had always been *high*. High. High. High. Now I was low, low, low. And dropping, even though I'd been woken up.

The Cardiologist arrived. His decision was swift and obvious. He switched the external pacemaker on and set it at 60bpm. The situation immediately resolved itself and my HR monitor was confirming the new, higher, steadier rate of 60bpm.

Once again, I was told this sort of thing wasn't unusual, which is exactly why the pacemaker wires are attached to the heart, during the operating procedure. That seemed to make sense. Although, my thoughts turned to ponder a whole series of questions:

- Why was this happening 11-12 days after the operation, when everything had been going so well?
- Is my issue now managing an intermittently low heart rate?
- Will the periods of high heart rate have gone away now the low rate issue has surfaced?
- What's causing this?
- How long will it last?
- Will it ever stop?
- Am I safe?

The last one is the shortest question but by far carried the most weight.

I levelled these questions at No.2 and his No.2 when they did their rounds the following morning. Not a great deal of clarity came back apart from the answer to the last question, which was, 'Absolutely. The pacemaker will ensure your heart rate won't drop to a critical level.'

Well, that was great, except I kind of meant, 'Am I safe if just left alone and flying solo?'

The response was what felt like a fudged answer. 'We're going to be monitoring you.' Which, when you're highly anxious, can sound remarkably like, *doing nothing*.

This wasn't true as, after a few hours, I was taken off the pacemaker to see how my heart was performing, unaided, which turned out to be fine. They also arranged to have a 24-hour ECG monitor fitted (known as a tape) which would be set up later that day. This would provide more detailed information on the electrical activity of my heart.

For the rest of the day, I was relieved my heart rate hadn't crashed like the value of a Rolf Harris art collection. Unfortunately though, there were a couple more pockets of a few hours, where we were back at 150. The 24-hour ECG was fitted after these two episodes, so didn't capture them. I was polarised about this. I wanted to get to the bottom of the issue but wasn't keen to have bad news confirmed. My thinking was, if there were no more arsey-hearty issues, captured on the ECG, then the medical team would declare all the previous episodes as blips, and that I was once again, an A-student in the art of recovery.

Such hopes were short-lived when I was woken in the early hours. Two nurses and a Cardiologist were already by my bed. The nurses had been monitoring my heart rate as, once again, it had dropped and was bottom-feeding at around 30. By now, I knew the script. The pacer was switched on and set at 60; the nurses went back to their station; the Grande Fromage disappeared back to his bunker and I went back to sleep. I was beginning to feel tired of worrying. I was tired of being in hospital. I was tired of setbacks. The novelty of this all-inclusive resort was wearing thin.

The next day, a familiar face walked into my room. Well, he was familiar to me. Although, I could tell he didn't recognise me, not straight away at least. It was Doc Swagger, who'd failed in his show-boating attempts to get an *Art Line* into my arm. Well, to be completely accurate, it'd been both arms. Twice. He was there to review recent events and to set up the 24-hour ECG.

He was empathising with me; telling me what a pain it was that my heart rate had started messing around like this. In line with all previous medical commentary, he was reassuring me that periods of rapid heart rate weren't uncommon after a CABG, but the sudden lower rates were a little more so. I'd become tired of hearing how being violently shaken from the inside was normal following my kind of procedure. Normal unless you're the one being violently shaken. In which case it's shittingly abnormal. But he had my attention with the second part of his statement.

I enquired about how low my heart rate might drop and how worried I should be. It was an interesting answer but delivered in a familiar manner.

'Ah don't b'worried – w'ill keep yer safe. But ar 'preciate its jes a fackin' pain in th'arse fer yer if ye'v to hev a pacemaker fitted... Ah sorry – ar relly sh'd watch m' language. Ar apologise if arv offended ye...'

I felt a cauldron of emotion and it wasn't the language. But most certainly, at the content. My reply was more than tainted with it.

'No offence taken. But I'm about 30 years younger than some people on this ward so if you talk like that in front of them, there's a fair fucking chance they might have something to say about it.'

There was a beat as he looked at me, then smiled and put his hands up in acknowledgement. 'No... yer right. Ar do apologise. But hey, it's you. Didn't ar see you in ICU?'

'You did.'

'Yer lookin' so much better. Ar did nae recognise yer wi the glasses on.'

'Well apart from my heart rate bouncing around, I'm feeling a lot better. But... what's this about a pacemaker?'

He could see the shock all over my face. 'Oh, arm no sayin that'll def'nitly 'appen but as no one talk'd to yer 'bout this?'

'Nope.'

'Arr... ok, well this tape wi' tell us a lot but ar suspect that yer ave Tachy Brady syndrome.'

'Whaty Whaty? What syndrome?'

'It's short fer tachycardia-bradycardia syndrome. Don't b'alarmed. It jes means tha sometimes yer heart goes too fast – the tachy – an sometimes it goes too slow – the brady. But notin' is decided. Let's jes see wha the tape picks up.'

Throughout the conversation, he was attaching sticky pads to my torso, connecting wires between them and the small recorder, and setting it up to capture my heart's activity over the next 24 hours. Once finished, he couldn't have got out of the room any quicker. He must have felt as if he'd walked into a minefield. But then had thrown a few grenades around anyway, just for good measure.

My overriding emotion was anger. I'd like to say frustration but based on the language coming out of my mouth, I think it was much closer to anger. What the actual fuck was going on? The word *pacemaker* had been used, in the context of me. Yeah, yeah... *'It'll no def'nitly 'appen,'* but even bringing it up as a possibility, in relation to me? It was bang out of order. And this was why it was bang out of order: a pacemaker is for old people. More than that - it's for decrepit old people. People whose hearts are blobs - just lumps of pulsating jelly. People who, if they didn't have their pacemaker, would descend into a gasping, convulsing demise even attempting to wipe their own arse. Having a pacemaker is literally like being plugged into a car battery. Not only that, a pacemaker restricts activity. There's no hill walking or cycling. Forget it. I doubt if even a hot & spicy pizza would be allowed for fear of flatlining.

*Pacemaker*. I couldn't get the word out of my head.

FFS. I couldn't bear the thought of this being me. If this is what the future entailed, I wasn't interested. Not that I even accepted it *was* my future. If it was even suggested, they could fuck right off.

They were going to have to do better than that. Try harder. Come up with a better solution. Something more fitting for a man of my age. For a man of my athletic prowess. Well, maybe best not to dwell on that too much, but more fitting of the athletic prowess I aspired to.

It wasn't that I hadn't been made aware of the potential for this to happen. Mr D had raised the possibility of a post-operative pace-maker when going through the consent form. But the quoted odds were 1/20. 5%. If I backed a 20-1 horse at Betfred, I'd never expect a payout. I'd also seen a couple of patients on the ward being told they needed pacemakers, just a few days after their operations. But those guys must have been in their ninth decade. Not fit young things like me, who'd be wanting to do all kinds of manly, athletic stuff.

I was absolutely livid.

Livid because of the way it was being considered behind the scenes as a possible, acceptable outcome, without even discussing it with me. Livid because frankly, I wasn't prepared to accept it and have activity options in my new life, my second life, ripped away from me. But the thing which made me most livid; the thing at the heart of my rage; was the absolute certainty with which I knew, *I just knew*, that this fucking awful thing *was* going to happen to me, that I wouldn't be able to stop it, and that I had no choice but to force myself to accept it. I didn't have to wait for any results from a tape, or for Doctors to rub their chins as they deliberated over the data.

It was inevitable. So, the sooner I wrapped my head around it, the better. That's what hurt the most. Accepting that, to move off that particular square in this shitty Jumanji game I never wanted to play, I'd have to take more shit to live a compromised future life.

And I want to be clear here, I wasn't in the least bit feeling sorry for myself. It was genuine anger that the activity levels I'd wanted to get back to, were now just going to be dreams once this thing was fitted. It'd be like living life with a handbrake on. What's more, if I knew it, other people would know it too:

'Poor bastard – I used to have a beer with him on a hill walk.'

'Poor bastard – I cycled with him from London to Paris.'

'Poor bastard – I ran half marathons with him.'

This future life: just a watercolour of what could have been, was light years away from the appetite I'd built up for the prospect of a second life. The second life wasn't about ripping up the first, it was about refining it; making improvements, reaping greater enjoyment, creating more joy... I was just waiting to realise how I was going to achieve it all. But now it appeared my second life would just be a weaker, diluted version of the first. So not really a second life at all. More like a half-life.

With that, I got my iPad out and furiously Googled pacemakers, hoping that super fit, speed-setting, middle-distance runners didn't come up as the first hits.

# 26

# The Shitometer

*"The problem is not the problem.*
*The problem is your attitude about the problem."*
**Captain Jack Sparrow**

I knew I'd need an informed conversation with Karina, as this news would be a shock to her too. Although I hadn't used the term *second life* by that stage with her, we'd both agreed we should use this as an opportunity to make changes in our lives. Particularly around my work-life balance. Sharing this latest development was going to be a tough conversation.

My first port of call was the British Heart Foundation site. Thankfully they seemed to know a tad more about these things than I did, as there was an impressive amount of information, including case studies. They're always going to put the poster boys and girls on this sort of site, but it was quite a relief to see a) not everyone looked recently exhumed, and b) they looked as though they could all do more than merely communicate via blinking.

It turns out having a pacemaker wasn't quite what I'd imagined. From what I could see, people still seemed to be able to work, rest and play as usual and the pacemaker wasn't a mobile substitute for plugging your heart into the mains, just to make it beat.

Who would have thought it?

Even after only a few minutes of skimming through various case studies, it was beginning to look like my reputation as a hill-walking, cycling, adventure-seeking, shagging machine, could possibly survive this bump in the road, intact. Far from putting the brakes on my output and activity, it'd be nothing more than a safety net, only kicking in if my heart rate went below a pre-set rate. It had only dipped overnight so depending on the set rate, this is probably the only time a device would pace.

I had lots of questions, naturally. Questions about the type of pacemaker, the fitting of it, potential infection from the procedure, battery life (so when I'd need another procedure), situations to avoid such as airport scanners... but these felt emotionally more manageable than being turned into an old man, 30 years ahead of time. This was good news; it strangely felt like another win.

*Any win's a win – and we take them all.*

It was more than *any old win*. Much more. It was a big win. If having a pacemaker made me safe from a sudden drop in heart rate (especially when I wasn't even conscious to know about it) and it didn't limit my activity in any way, then it was a no brainer. There was only an upside, so it was a massive win. Don't get me wrong, I still didn't want it to happen. I didn't want the procedure. I didn't want to think of my heart needing this *just in case* safety net, to avoid dropping through the floor overnight. But if having a pacemaker had no impact on my woken life and was only doing a job when I was asleep, then I was comfortable with that. I could accept it.

It was bizarre. I felt proud of myself for getting my head around it before it had even been properly discussed or decided that I needed one. Jumping to my worst fears seemed to have inoculated me against what was a much tamer reality. There's so much about our health that we can't control. There's plenty we can *influence*, but a total lack of control can easily cause anxiety and upset, which affects our mental and physical well-being. And the spiral continues. But I'd regained just a little bit of control. Not in terms of outcome, but in terms of how I'd mentally prepared for that potential outcome.

I'd become used to very little happening over the weekends. It's not so much that they operate on a skeletal crew (although they often do), more like a reluctant one. If decisions can be deferred to weekdays, they tend to be. If decisions don't have to be proactively made, they aren't. If a reactive decision is needed to a patient's situation, then naturally it's made, but generally, non-critical decisions were avoided between Friday evening and Monday morning. So, it was quite a surprise on Sunday morning when I was visited by a Cardiologist I'd not seen before, telling me she'd reviewed the report from my 24-hour ECG and confirmed I appeared to have developed Tachy-Brady Syndrome. What she couldn't say with confidence was whether this would be a permanent situation.

However, her recommendation was to manage the situation through a combination of meds for the higher rate and a pacemaker for the lower rate. Always thinking ahead, I asked about the battery life. I really didn't want to be going through this every few years. I was told, depending on use, 8-10 years and as technology developed, batteries would improve. I could live with that.

She thought the PM (naturally there's an abbreviation) would be fitted on Wednesday and also said Gordon would be on call the following day and she'd ask him to drop in.

Since Doc Swagger had first mentioned the word, not only had I got my head around it, I'd also had so many more phases of high and low heart rate. As such, it was very clear a solution of some sort was needed. This *Whaty-Whaty* syndrome wasn't going to go away all by itself. After my last hospital discharge, I wasn't going to be leaving the building until they'd decided I was safe. Until *I* felt safe, myself. And I wasn't going to be safe until this power pack was fitted.

A bit like Iron Man. Kind of.

By the time Gordon visited the following day, I'd formed a whole raft of questions, but I led with the one that weighed most heavily on my mind: taking into account the remodelling carried out on my heart; once I'd had the PM fitted and my meds were finalised to manage the higher rate, would I be *just* as likely as a bloke of my age to have a heart attack or another cardiac arrest? Or would I still always have a *higher* chance of that happening?

It was a long way of asking – is this likely to happen to me again? The Police frontman looked at me with curiosity and almost a hint of disbelief. I'll never forget his response.

'No, no, you don't understand. You have a much *less* chance of anything like this happening again. It took 50 years to get here. Think of it as your heart having had a full service. The blood supply is running smoothly; the valve repair is working well; the AF should disappear altogether and you're on preventative meds.'

I was about to ask about the pacemaker, but he hadn't finished. 'I know it must have been disappointing to learn about the pacemaker, but we have to make sure that you're safe. To be honest, in terms of what pacemakers can do, yours will be doing very little. It'll be a 2-wire model. Think of it as some pacemakers being Skodas and some being Formula One cars. Both do their jobs perfectly well, but one demands more performance. Yours will be more Skoda.'

This was Gordon at his very best. Calming, reassuring and with the bedside manner of Sting. He was on his A-game. I wanted to hug him. He could see the relief in my face as I said, 'At first, I was bothered about the pacemaker, but not now. It's the future I'm worried about. I can't go through all this again. Me or my family. So... what you're saying is... I'm in a better cardiac place than most other 50-year-old blokes?'

Gordon understood where I was coming from and wasn't finished with his soothing words.

'Look - I know your heart better than I know my own. There are walking time bombs out there - your age, younger and older. Your heart is running clear. And you're on watch. You'll have some early reviews, which will then become annual, and we'll keep an eye on your meds to make sure they're only doing what they're supposed to do and no more. The pacemaker will also be checked annually and that in itself can provide a lot of useful data.'

He was literally lifting weights from my shoulders.

'I just want to get back out being active,' I replied, like a broken record. But it was true. The thought of having the choice of any given activity taken away from me was really frightening. Even if I wouldn't necessarily have chosen to do that given activity. It must have sounded out of place with how I looked. By then, I was emaciated. My shorts and t-shirt were hanging off me, my arms and legs were like bits of string dangling out of those baggy clothes and I still had a drain tube and wires stitched into me.

'Karl, you've been so positive and optimistic throughout this whole process, it's been incredible. I spend most of my life trying to encourage people to be more active, so when I come across someone like you who's already motivated to be active, I do everything I possibly can to get them back to where they want to be – and beyond. I know you want to be back on your bike and walking in the hills and you will be. But everything needs to be built up slowly.'

I was wondering how slow, slowly would be. He expanded.

'I know how much the activity side of things means to you, but you're going to have to be gentle and kind to yourself. You'll need to be patient with progress. Once you leave hospital, you'll feel the pace of physical improvement slow down. But then there's the mental side too. Sometimes you'll be ahead mentally and other times your body will be ahead. You might feel a bit down, either about progress or just reflecting on what's happened. All of this is normal and part of the whole recovery process. But if you begin to feel weighed down emotionally, then we can help with that too. There are people who we can arrange for you to talk to.'

'I think I'm OK at the moment,' I replied, probably not that convincingly. But then, the person affected is usually the last to know.

'OK, but after everything you've been through, sometimes it can take a while for the body and mind to get back into step.'

The conversation pretty much wrapped up after that. I thanked him for everything he'd done, and he said he'd probably not see me again before I was discharged but wished me luck and left the room.

He was right – I didn't see him again, but that conversation will stay with me for the rest of my life. With the relief, came the emotion. That conversation was just the tonic I'd needed at that point in time, and he hadn't even reached for his prescription pad.

Shortly after Gordon's visit, two mates came into the ward to see me. I said I'd meet them in the hospital corridor, just for a change of scenery and to stretch my legs. As I walked up, they started laughing.

'What?' I said, 'good to see you too.'

'Sorry mate, but that's the worst European away football strip ever,' one of them said.

I looked down and they were right. I was wearing green, tight, knee-high compression socks, my blue cargo pants, and a bright pink t-shirt. I barely filled any of them. It wasn't a great look. They weren't fully up to speed with what had happened to me, so I told them as succinctly as possible, and they were visibly shocked.

One of them was a Police Sergeant and he said that plenty of his colleagues have had to deliver CPR over the years. He also confirmed just how challenging it was to get a positive outcome. If trained professionals would struggle to get a result with CPR, how on earth had

Karina managed to do it? Statistically, I shouldn't have been there. The thought was beginning to weigh on me. The visit was a lot more banter-full and appreciated than it sounds, but it did get me thinking about the second life thing again, or more specifically, something about it that should be different.

There's a Keynote Speaker we'd worked with many times called Paul McGee. He's a Professor, author, speaker, coach, trainer – his first big-selling book and the core of his delivery is around SUMO: Shut Up & Move On. He's known as The SUMO Guy and has a very down to earth and easy to understand delivery and always received masses of positive feedback from attendees.

As you might expect, one of the core aspects of Shutting Up & Moving On is to try and keep things in perspective, especially all the annoying little things in life. Just *shut up and move on.*

Paul came up with a beautifully simple but incredibly powerful way of approaching life's challenges, no matter what the size. He'd say that when a problem or challenge presents itself, imagine a scale of 1 to 10, where 1 is not much at all and 10 will result in death, or at least is life-threatening; and then ask, *where does this problem lie?* All too often, we'd feel like something was a 7, but when you stop and really think about it, it might be nearer a 3... a 4 at tops. Being stuck in traffic and being late for a meeting can feel like a stressful 7 but it surely couldn't be 3 off life-threatening? So, it might be nearer a 3 or 4. Even if it's an important meeting, delays happen to everyone from time to time, so other people tend to be quite forgiving. In fact, most problems or challenges tend to slide to that side of the scale when you really think about them.

I'd always liked that tool. I'm not saying I was always brilliant at applying it. It's hard to alter your automatic, often default reaction, especially if someone cuts you up on the road or you've been trying to buy gig tickets on a website that keeps freezing – and then they're suddenly sold out.

But it got me thinking. What if I adjusted the scale?

What if, when gauging a problem or *bad stuff*, 1 was not much at all, but 10 became, *I'm already dead*.

Not life-threatening, but actually... dead.

How would everything else in life compare? All the bad shit, I mean. I'd experienced a 10.

Compared to that 10, everything else had to rank lower. So, did that mean the worst thing that could ever happen to me personally, had already happened? Very possibly.

I mean, it would be awful if a family member became terminally ill or had life-changing injuries. I may have to make up an 11 in those situations – I don't know. But to me personally, being dead will have been the worst thing that had happened, in my life. Which doesn't even make sense as a sentence.

Losing my income? Not as bad at being dead.

Becoming bankrupt? Nope, I know a few of those and they're still very much better off than being dead.

Getting divorced? Devastating – but it happens in almost 50% of marriages. People survive.

This was a serious amount of perspective unfolding. My thinking went on.

It felt like 10 (I'm dead), was such an outlier and everything and anything between 1 (not much at all) and 9 (life-threatening), was skewed massively to the far left of that scale. So, if you were to try to put the scale on this page, 1-9 would be shoved into the width of a postage stamp on the far-left hand side and 10 would be far over to the right, almost in the next postcode. Such is the scale of the problem, compared to all your other problems, when you're dead.

This 1-10 scale I rebranded as *The Shitometer*.

There's another brilliant Speaker we've worked with, almost every year of my event company's existence, sometimes a few times a year called Damian Hughes. He's another Professor, an organisational psychologist who specialises in building winning cultures with sports teams and athletes but also works quite closely with businesses. He's now also the co-host of the brilliant, award-winning High Performance Podcast with Jake Humphrey. (Look it up - you won't regret it.) He's got this innate skill of seeing the strengths and weaknesses of a situation or organisation and an encyclopaedic knowledge of psychological research, cultural references and sporting anecdotes. I'd always got on with him really well and when he'd heard I was in hospital, he'd sent a hamper full of lovely goodies which helped build me back up, no end. When I was back on civvy street, I phoned him to thank him for the hamper. We had a long chat and I told him in more detail what had happened to me, how Karina had saved my life and also about my new barometer - The Shitometer. My *not much at all* to *I'm dead* scale. (I know, I know – it's not mine, I just rebranded it.) I shared that my Shitometer was telling me that the worst had already happened.

'You know what that is?' he said.

'No. What?'

'That's your Superpower. You've got the perspective to judge life's challenges and worries against the ultimate worst outcome - and that's already happened. Yet here you are, talking to me. If you can apply and harness that level of control, you do realise you can go through the rest of your life, without ever worrying about anything too much, ever again? When it comes to decision making, I'd call that a Superpower, wouldn't you?'

'Fuck – I'd not thought of it that way.'

'That's quite a liberating thought, isn't it?'

It certainly was. And one I vowed to integrate into this second life of mine. I'd never had a Superpower before – so that had to be another massive win. And at that point, I started to Google capes.

On the Tuesday afternoon, a nurse casually stuck her head around my door and asked, 'Oh Karl, is it OK if we move you onto the ward? We've got a really poorly guy coming in and we'll need to keep a close eye on him.'

It wasn't really a question, was it? It was a tell. An instruction. But what could I say?

'Yea of course – no problem. How long have I got?'

'About an hour.'

'No worries, I'll pack all my stuff together,' I replied. Far too happily.

FFS! I loved having my own room! Now I'll have to talk to and listen to strangers. Not to mention Karina and I having to reign in vocalising our observations. I felt an inner, mini-rant brewing.

Superpower... Superpower... on a scale of 1 to 10, where does this problem lie?

Well, as problems go, this one went, in a flash. Because on reflection, this wasn't a problem at all. This was a great sign that someone, somewhere had decided my progress warranted a less watchful eye. This was not a problem. This was another win.

Within the hour, I was ensconced on the ward, in an end bed (thumbs up), next to the window (double thumbs up) and had already had a chat with three of the other blokes in my bay. One of them was a Postman and he was worried about having to go back to his eight-mile, hilly, round. Another one was self-employed and was worried about not having any sick pay, so knew he'd have to get back to work sooner rather than later. The final guy was recovering from having an infection following a heart valve replacement. There was another guy, fast asleep, ashen looking, oxygen mask on, having recently had a severe heart attack. The final bed was empty.

I was thankful not to have been in any of their situations. I really did feel quite fortunate and privileged not to be burdened by those kinds of work issues and the pressure that can bring, or, as ridiculous as it sounds, by dire health issues, such as some of theirs.

Even taking the 1-10, Diddly-to-Death Shitometer out of it; no matter how much shit you think you have on your plate or in your life, you can often find that shit is relative. Someone else would love to have your shit, given the chance. But that's the problem with shit, isn't it? Sometimes even a small amount can feel overpowering and stink like hell.

# 27

# The Great Escape

*"Strength doesn't come from winning. Your struggles develop your strengths. When you go through hardships and decide not to surrender, that is strength."*
**Arnold Schwarzenegger**

Wednesday 29<sup>th</sup> May 2019 – Pacemaker Fitting Day.

*Nil By Mouth* was written on the whiteboard to the side of my bed at 11am and I was gowned up by 2pm. I'd been told I'd be going into theatre at about 3pm but it ended up being nearer 4pm. That's quite a long time without liquids. Especially if someone needs to find a vein for a cannula and the patient's blood pressure has dropped due to dehydration. A couple of male nurses had a couple of stabs each (literally) and then a Junior Doctor had a couple more stabs and finally succeeded. It crossed my mind as to whether their success rate would increase if, after failing, I had a go on them, and we alternated like Russian Roulette. Or perhaps if they invested in a vein-finder, which apparently, is a thing.

I left Karina on the ward, as I took my place on the all too familiar blue wheelchair and was trundled off to theatre. There was something eerily familiar about the surroundings. I stepped up onto the operating table, had the side panels slotted in, a heated blanket put over me and I was given a mild sedative through the cannula. The

Cardiologist then introduced himself and sat on a stool just to the left of my shoulder. It was a few minutes before any further conversation was directed at me, although there had been plenty of chatter. When the Cardiologist next spoke directly to me, it was to tell me that he was about to administer the local anaesthetic and I should let him know if I could feel anything.

What I felt was shit-scared when I saw the size of the needle. I'd had a few injections in my time and in no way do I have any phobia of needles, but this bad boy was the Daddy of them all. Somehow though, I don't think he was interested in that kind of feeling. He pressed the needle against the skin just below my left collar bone. I felt the contact and the pop through the skin but nothing more, so all was good. He got on with his work and I got on with mine. He may have been inserting the wires and putting them in position. I couldn't be sure. There were shades of the Angiogram in that there was a lot of looking at a large screen and exchanges of English words which meant nothing to me. My job was to lay as still as possible and take myself off to my happy place, which at that point in time, was anywhere in the World, outside of those theatre doors. I just happened to have selected a quiet beach by the village of Humberston, where I grew up.

I was a four-year-old, building a massive sandcastle with my brother when I was suddenly distracted by somebody telling me they were going to administer some more anaesthetic. Not what my four-year-old self wanted to hear, so it must have been aimed at my 50-year-old self. Although to be fair, my 50-year-old self wasn't that keen on hearing it either. Nonetheless, same procedure; needle on the skin, pressure applied, but no pain. Then another – that one did make me wince a little. And another. Yep that was definitely more painful and felt deeper. I fed this back, received an apology, and was told we'd wait a few minutes for the local to take full effect.

It's entirely possible they waited for a few minutes, but to me, it felt like he only waited until he'd finished the sentence. It was at that point I saw the scalpel and had to turn away. Needles - even the Daddy of - I can handle, but the mental image of that thin sliver of metal separating my skin and muscle? No. That, and the anticipation of the pain that would accompany it. No, no, no. Many times, no. This was one of those moments when only the scrunched-up insides of your eyelids can give you a modicum of comfort.

But the pain didn't come. I didn't even feel the contact with my skin. The relief was immense. I think I may have stopped breathing as I'd braced for impact, so let out quite a big sigh when I realised that bit was over.

But then the tugging started.

It felt like my shoulder area was being thrust towards my feet, but not from being pushed externally, from the top, but being pulled from somewhere within. Next was the sound and sensation of tearing, and I felt a sharp sting in the area he was working. I let out some poorly muted primaeval sound.

'I'm sorry, I'm just making the pocket,' was the reply, as another thrust generated another tearing sound. It wasn't the kind of sound you could hear through your ears; more like a resonance through the body as tissue was being separated from tissue. A noise, universally associated with pain, left my lips.

'Can you feel that?' the Cardiologist asked incredulously. We had a breakthrough.

'Yeh,' I said, possibly the fastest I'd ever said it.

'Really? Oh, I'm sorry. You shouldn't be able to feel a thing. I'll administer some more anaesthetic.'

Out came the Daddy again, which this time was no longer scary at all. Now it was my best friend. In it plunged, delivering its magic nectar to take me away from this moment in time and space. A few minutes were allowed to pass. The Cardiologist filled them with small talk to his team. I filled them by trying to regain control of my breathing concentrating on not vomiting.

He continued. I could still hear the ripping sound from within my own body, but the pain was fully gone. I accepted the compromise and some form of relaxation followed.

I didn't feel the device being placed into *the pocket*, but I did feel it being stitched in position. There was no associated pain, but I could feel the Cardiologist's arms shaking as he strained to ensure whatever knot he was tying on each suture, was tighter than a gnat's chuff. There were a few of these super-duper strained knots put in place, followed by some cleaning and a light spreading of glue over the wound and a gauze dressing. And that was it. The whole process took around 45 minutes. See you again in about 10 years.

I was taken back to the ward, and I felt surprisingly spritely. I had no pain at all in the collar bone area and was by that time, about 5:15pm, prepared to eat a buttered brick. I scoffed whatever was on offer from the hospital dinner rounds and Karina also brought me some sandwiches and fruit, which I inhaled.

I'd been told the pacemaker would be checked by a Specialist the following day and I wasn't to raise my left arm above my shoulder for six weeks. This was to avoid *lead displacement* which I seriously wanted to avoid. The thought of accidentally tugging one or both leads out of position on my heart and having to go through any corrective measures filled me with fear. So, whilst the prescribed restriction of movement did concern me a little (as I hadn't yet regained full mobility in my left shoulder following the CABG), the alternative of further repair work, was not an option. As such, I heeded this instruction rigidly. With possibly a little too much emphasis on the *rigidly*.

The close of that day was my 22nd night in hospital during that stay. Prior to that, I'd spent a further 20 nights across the two hospitals. A total of 42 nights with a cardiac arrest and a bypass operation in the middle. As Freddie would have said, 'It's been no bed of roses.' It was beginning to wear thin. For everyone.

I was, by that stage intensely bored, and fed up with my life and existence being compromised so much. I was tired of being the focus of attention in my immediate world. And my immediate world felt exactly the same. More so than me.

Karina was exhausted. She'd visited me every day, sometimes twice a day, making a one hour round trip each time. But that's just the driving. Then there's the getting ready, gathering stuff to bring in (from home or shops), finding the parking space, the walk to the ward (which in that hospital could generate your daily 10k steps on its own) before you even get to managing the emotional rollercoaster we were on and everything she'd seen and been through.

There was also the minor issue of managing the boys. The stress of A' levels, school exams and general coursework to be kept on top of. Rugby training and matches for both, which also meant attending the matches. There was kickboxing training to get to and from. And again, this is all before you even get to help them manage their own emotions. Teenagers are not known for proactively sharing their thoughts, especially troubled thoughts. It takes a Specialist, highly trained, with years of experience in looking for clues, alert to non-verbal communication and reading between the lines, to be able to interpret what's going on below the surface. That Specialist is called a Parent. Even then, we often get it wrong and misjudge a situation.

Let's not forget running the home: meal planning, food shopping, meal prep, keeping on top of the laundry (gathering, washing, drying and on rare occasions, even ironing), keeping the house clean, the constant running battle with the dishwasher...

But beyond all the above, I'm sure the most demanding aspect of my six-week secondment to the NHS, was having to manage her own emotions and holding it all together. All I did was lay there, sit there or wander around, all day long.

I don't know how she did it. Her Mum was a godsend and had moved in pretty much as soon as I was admitted the second time, which was a massive help and even bigger comfort. And Sarah too played an invaluable role in helping keep the emotional demons away.

We were also blessed with a never-ending supply of support from friends. Everyone seemed to be rallying to our cause. Homemade meals were brought round, the boys were brought to hospital, lifts were offered for sports activities, they were taken on a camping trip as well as countless other activities. Mostly Karina didn't even ask. Sometimes, help was offered, but mostly, our lovely friends just stepped in, took control, and initiated support. You all know who you are and our whole family will be forever grateful.

But even so, never underestimate the resilience required by those supporting those who are in hospital for an extended spell. Their mental strength is far deeper, wider, and more elastic than those lounging around inside. But by the end of that day, there wasn't much depth, width or elasticity left. Karina was truly exhausted, and I completely understood. I was merely very fed up.

We'd both latched on to the notion of *Any Win's A Win - And We Take Them All*. It'd become a mantra over the previous couple of weeks. We fed off it. We looked out for the wins. Anything at all to confirm we were moving forward and making progress, no matter how slowly. But what we really needed to offset the exhaustion, was a big win. And by then, in our minds, the only thing that would qualify as a big win, was to be allowed home.

The following day proved to be significant in so many ways. Firstly, I woke up to discover I was in a huge amount of pain. The PM wound and surrounding area were harbouring a deep, intense, internal ache. The kind of pain that can't be ignored and leaves you feeling demented. The first nurse of the day appeared ready for this reaction and gave me two tablets as soon as I woke up. So started a regular diet of high dosage Co-codamol. I can confirm they are both rapid and excellent relievers of pain - and not a grasshopper in sight. I wholeheartedly recommend them.

A little later that morning, the PM Specialist signed off their handiwork and I was told I wouldn't be seen again until October. Another win. One which I hoped was building up to the ultimate big win.

Just after lunch, Mr D arrived by my bed along with two other Doctors, although it was mildly disappointing that the man I'd come to know as 'No.2', his right-hand man, was standing on his left. I'm going to have to work on my OCD.

The usual questions were asked; he checked my notes and read the update from the PM Specialist; examined my various wounds and then caught me totally off guard. 'You know Karl, I think it's about time we allowed you to finish your recovery at home.'

And just like that, the win we'd been seeking, was delivered. I was so excited. I thrust my hand out, over-vigorously shook his hand and was all teethy smiles. I was that bloke on a politician's walkabout. The one where the bloke thinks the politician is his best mate and the politician wants that brief second in time captured on camera as proof of popularity but has already mentally moved on before the bloke has finished shaking hands. Yup. I was he.

Not that Mr D sought popularity. He only sought results. Given how everything had unravelled the last time I was discharged, I was confident in his confidence, in sending me home.

I was told the nurses would remove the external pacing wires and the drain, and he'd need to raise a prescription with the Pharmacy Dept for meds to take home, but I should be on my way the following day, Friday. Home for the weekend. Karina cried when I told her the news. And then I cried. That phase of our lives was nearly over.

At about 2pm a nurse came to remove the external pacing wires. Although on reflection, using the word 'remove' is only really 50% true. There were four wires in total, two atrial and two ventricular. To this day, the two atrial wires are still inside me and will be for the rest of my life. Usually, all four wires are pulled out but for some reason, Mr D always requested his patients' atrial wires are only cut. Apparently, he was unique in this approach, amongst surgeons at that hospital. I made a mental note to raise it with him when we next discussed cardio-thoracic surgical techniques.

That was the penultimate win, leaving only the drain as the final item still plumbed into me. The good news was there'd been no gunky liquid appearing in the drain bottle since it'd been changed ten days prior. Even the original bottle hadn't managed to syphon much maroon mucus from my chest for the two or three days before it'd been replaced.

However, it was kept in place for another hour or two to see if it picked anything up from the removal of the ventricular wires. It made sense, I suppose, but was a little frustrating. I wanted to kill the game off there and then but apparently, we were going into extra time.

My frustration was short-lived, as within 90 minutes the nurse was back to remove the drain. This was the final shackle keeping me in hospital. Losing it was as symbolic as it was a physical acknowledgement, that this stage of my recovery was coming to an end. But I knew to get there, I'd have to endure a few more seconds of organ suction. Two words a male wouldn't usually preface with *endure*.

I was familiar with the routine and braced for the big finale but either my body was so much stronger by then, or the nurse was bloody good (possibly both), but it was all over with one swift pain-free tug.

The final win. Freedom from my shackles. I almost couldn't sleep that night with the excitement of going home the following day. That, and the pain from the PM wound.

Friday 30th May – my final day in hospital. I'd been there every day throughout May, albeit with an 18-hour hiatus between the 7th and 8th, as well as 14 nights in April. I'd been in the wilderness for 43 nights and 44 days. I had bested JC's desert walk by four whole days. In no way am I saying this makes me better than he. I'm just observing the facts.

I was dressed and packed, ready for a mid-morning departure. All I needed was a Pharmacist to drop off my new medication and I would be homeward bound. For the second time. Eventually, my meds arrived at about 4pm. The intervening time was like having your return flight from a holiday delayed and having to wait, with your bags, tired and fed up, for news of your departure.

Having been in hospital for so long, I felt uncomfortable not saying *thanks and goodbye* to every member of the team who'd helped me over those weeks. But similar to when I left SLI ICU, many who had cared for me weren't on shift and nearly all who were on shift, were tied up with patients. So, we thanked those we saw en route to the ward exit but made no detours. I had a return journey to complete and I wasn't going to mess it up. Each pause on the way to the main exit ran the risk of someone, somewhere realising they'd made a gargantuan mistake and that, unfortunately, I should really be back enjoying hospital food for a good while yet.

It was a joy to stand outside the hospital, once we'd cleared all the hacking, diabetic, amputee smokers, sponsored by RIZLA. I waited at the edge of the car park as Karina collected the car and brought it around. I couldn't have a seatbelt over my left shoulder due to the pain of the PM wound, so sat in the passenger seat behind Karina. Even then, I also wedged a pillow between the seat belt and my body to protect my chest wound. It was a surreal image, but a significant one. After everything we'd all gone through, I'd always thought I'd feel elated during that moment, finally achieving the big win we had coveted so much - going home. But elation seemed a far cry from how I was feeling. I'd become Mr Daisy and as my chauffeur pulled us away from the car park, for the first time since my pre-op shave, I felt a sense of sadness... for me. For having had to go through it all. I'd felt sad for Karina and the boys countless times, but not really for myself, until that point. But then at least I was around to feel sad. Even buried deep within sadness, there's a win.

# 28

# The Sign Off

*"I always get to where I'm going
by walking away from where I have been."*
**Winnie the Pooh**

I didn't do too much that first weekend. I was some way off actively filling my newfound freedom. The one stand-out occurrence was on the Saturday morning. Three mates had generously given up part of their weekend to tidy our garden which had taken on primaeval properties. I was still in the bedroom in my jimmies when I heard a petrol strimmer and mower chug into life. I hadn't seen these mates for weeks so threw some random shorts and t-shirt on and went outside to catch up with them. Many months later, one told me he'd been shocked when he saw me. Apparently, I looked like a massively emaciated Frank Skinner (sorry Frank). Which is strange because I distinctly remember wanting to demonstrate how well I looked. Such is the power of perspective.

My escape from hospital was short-lived as I had to go back on the Monday to have my zip stitches removed and pick up more meds. It was no biggie really, yet once again my Spider-senses were tingling. Some prehistoric early warning system was telling me to remain vigilant for Sabre-toothed Tigers, bad-ass dudes from the neighbouring tribe or anyone approaching with a blue wheelchair saying, "There you are! Now sit down and we'll get you back to the ward..."

Having navigated the perma-Rizla-Brigade at the entrance, my readiness to rumble was still with me as we approached the ward where I'd spent so long and experienced so much. Even the hospital smell hit me afresh. Like it was suddenly new to me again, despite having been surrounded by it for weeks previously. I was genuinely apprehensive. It wasn't an overwhelming feeling, but it made itself known. I was barely talking and kept alert to anyone approaching with purpose. It was as if the power of the institution was greater than me and at will, I could be pulled back in by some NHS Death Star tractor beam. There was no reason on earth for this to happen, but I'd clearly become conditioned to the ways of the ward: if they look for something, they'll find something. In the end, you just want them to stop looking.

A nurse checked my wounds over, was happy with them and took the stitches out of the main zip. The glue on the PM wound was still very much attached and would be for a week or so, so no action required. There was no listening to my chest or taking blood pressure or any other searching for potential reasons to be re-admitted, which was a comfort. 'I'll be out of there in minutes,' I thought.

She then apologised and explained the Pharmacist still hadn't dropped my meds off. She'd already chased but would do so again. Outwardly I was swan calm. Inwardly, I was a covert Ops team, behind enemy lines, requiring immediate evac. It was another two hours before we left the ward. Two hours on a chronometer at least. I'd visibly aged by the time we'd got the meds and were back at the car.

Although not an overly enjoyable experience (despite my liberty never once being threatened), it offered up a moment for which I was grateful. I'd approached the Nurses' Station to chase up the

Pharmacist and realised I was standing next to the young male nurse who'd delivered the words of wisdom that had become integral to our thinking. I just dived straight in.

'Excuse me. You probably won't remember me. I'm Karl. Karl Perry. You transferred me from ICU to that room there almost three weeks back,' I enthused, far, far too gushingly.

'Oh, yea – hi. I think I remember you. How're you doing? You're looking well,' he said in a manner that suggested he had no recollection at all and was wondering whether to call Security. I ignored his diluted enthusiasm and ploughed on.

'Look, this is going to sound weird, but you said something to me that day. Something I'll never forget and I just want to thank you for it,' and I instinctively offered him my hand, which he instinctively took and shook, although clearly with an equal mix of curiosity and confusion.

'Really? You're welcome.' There was a brief beat. 'What did I say?'

'You said,' and I could feel my throat tightening up, 'you said... "any win's a win – and we take them all." And I know it sounds daft, but it really resonated with me, and I've tried to apply it ever since. And it just makes so much sense to me and... and... just thank you...'

Poor lad. He had an emotional, gushing, scrawny, middle-aged man in baggy clothes, he couldn't remember standing in front of him, attaching deep meaning to something he apparently said, but also, clearly couldn't remember saying.

'Well, it sounds like the kind of thing I'd say, so... I'm glad to have helped and that you're feeling so much better.'

I thanked him once again and the conversation wrapped itself up. We went our separate ways and I doubt and hope our paths will ever cross in a professional capacity, again. Even if they did, I'm not sure I'd recognise him after all this time. He certainly didn't recognise me after only three weeks, so I won't expect a tap on the shoulder any time soon. It just goes to show the impact our words can have on people, without us even realising. And that can work negatively too, so perhaps we should all tread a little lighter.

During the weeks and months that followed, apart from the top part of my chest wound opening into an ulcer-like sore which took six weeks to heal, the physical side of recovery went from strength to strength.

Shortly after discharge, I attended Cardiac Rehab; an eight-week gym course, aimed at rebuilding strength and stamina. I initially had my doubtful boots on as to whether attending would be worth it but was willing to give anything a go to speed up my return to normality. To my surprise, it was impressively beneficial. I didn't turn into Arnie overnight. That took some time. But I did discover I wasn't made of glass and it helped with the walking. And walk, we did.

I was out walking every day with Karina, usually to the local park and initially not particularly fast, but as the weeks went by, the walks grew longer, faster and we took in more of the slopes. It was summer and I wanted to be outside as much as possible, so that park became our best friend. There was always the incentive of a visit to the café, too. Oh God. I was turning into my Mother.

Looking back on that time, I have quite fond memories of my walks with Karina, and I know she does too. We obviously spent a lot of time talking and reflecting but also musing about the future. We both felt there had to be a restructuring in our lives, mine primarily. I needed to address the stress:happiness imbalance generated by the role I'd created for myself, in the company I'd founded and built. The tail was wagging the dog and it was hard to believe the imbalance hadn't contributed, on some level, to where I'd found myself on 8th May. It wasn't something that could be immediately addressed but during those walks, I really focussed on my earlier thinking whilst in hospital. Given the opportunity of this second life, there would be some changes made. Otherwise, what was the point of the opportunity?

Something which had to be addressed as a matter of urgency was the ability to dress myself. Not a skill you'd ever consider including on a CV, but quite a useful one, nonetheless. My left shoulder was still frozen. If anything, it'd become worse. Getting it to 45 degrees was an achievement, but the resistance caused teeth-clenching pain. This was beyond my finger walking exercises. I needed the help of a pro so visited a nearby Physio and paid to experience a great deal more pain.

During the initial consultation, it was mentioned I could have a series of injections to loosen my shoulder up. I went old school and opted for the hands-on approach. In a rare moment of maturity, I felt my body was already awash with drugs. If I could avoid adding to the cocktail, I should.

It'd be fair to say the Physio was quite petite in build, but I quickly discovered she had the strength of a UFC Champion as her hands pushed deep into my soft, toneless tissue. Her thumbs were made of an element yet to be discovered. She was always very smiley and laughed a lot. I cried a lot. It was an abusive relationship really. I should have walked away but stayed for the kids. (Mine. Not hers.) If I didn't get my shoulder fixed, I'd never be able to return to my Taxi-Dad duties. Gradually though, my tendons were reminded of their role in Team Pezza and after five sessions and plenty of homework, I was pretty much back to pre-operative movement. Yet another person to add to the growing team of people who'd either helped or were helping me get to a place somewhere close to normal. And yet another win. Never underestimate the privilege of being able to get dressed, unaided.

Mr D signed me off at the end of June with the caveat of not hitting the hills on my bike for another six months. I was gutted about that. Although I had no intention of cycling straight away, I'd hoped that by the end of August I would be, but reasoned it was a small price to pay in retaining my membership of the 8% Club. The sign off was a big win. A massive win. A milestone on my, our, recovery journey. Everything had hinged on Mr D being happy with his work and my progress because of it. Him giving me the green light meant the good ship *Normality* was in port and I'd been given a boarding pass. I can't lie, though. I was slightly disappointed he hadn't wanted to keep in touch after the rollercoaster journey we'd been on together. But then it's unreasonable to expect a heart surgeon to be pen pals with every patient he's had his hands in.

Before I'd even left hospital, I'd decided that once I had the all-clear, I'd pop back in with some goodies for the nurses and teams who'd looked after me. Specifically, I wanted to thank the Critical Care Unit for my time between admission and the operation, Nat and Anita in the ICU and the teams on the ward. Once again there was a sense of unease, returning to the scenes of so much physical and emotional trauma, but thankfully, less so this time. Possibly more of a recollection of the emotions than experiencing them again, although it's sometimes difficult to tell them apart.

Hardly anyone I wanted to see was on shift. I was so disappointed. I really wanted to share my appreciation to close the circle of my hospital journey. I was particularly disappointed with my trip to ICU. Nat was with a patient (I should have guessed) and Anita had recently left to go on Maternity Leave. I hadn't even noticed she was pregnant. Had that been down to the painkillers she'd been feeding me or an indication of where my focus had been? Probably a bit of both. Either way, that visit boxed off the hospitalisation stage of my recovery and I began to focus on new challenges.

# 29

## Seismic Shifts

*"Never do anything by halves if you want to get away with it.*
*Be outrageous. Go the whole hog."*

**Matilda**

I hadn't put much store on Gordon's references to the mental side of recovery, *'be patient... sometimes the mind will be ahead and sometimes it'll be the body.'* Doctors often speak in generalised terms because patients react in different ways, whether to procedures, medicines or in recovery. I understood that. He was covering all the ground he had to and quite rightly. But it didn't apply to me. I knew it wouldn't – I'd been so resilient in my work and personal life for decades – it was all I knew. Mentally I managed and I managed well. Notwithstanding the long periods of middle-of-night insomnia.

Perhaps because I was going to bed, healthy, if not yet fully recovered, in the same room where my body had stopped functioning, or maybe because I was no longer in hospital, but I truly believed I was over the worst of it. Although that said, I'd also begun to reflect on the 8% figure. Why had I fallen into that camp and not the other 92%? It's a colossal imbalance. What happened to create the outcome as it did? It's easy to say, 'Well Karina carried out the CPR as instructed, and we were very lucky.' Both of those factors are incredibly true. Karina had saved my life – for the second time. But that didn't address the magnitude of what had happened. And equally, what hadn't happened, which if it had, would have tilted the outcome the other way. I couldn't shake off the belief that, prior to the cardiac arrest, I would never have regarded myself as being that lucky. So, over the course of those early days and weeks of being at home, I began to mine down into what had to have happened, or not, for me to have made the 8%. It didn't make for easy thinking.

Firstly, Karina had to have been in the room with me. This was never a given. She could have been downstairs watching morning TV or on her phone, in the shower, or any other room in the house. Or, it might have been me in the shower, in the bathroom, downstairs...

What if Karina had taken longer to realise what was happening to me?

Then there's the phone. If a phone has been mislaid in our house, it's usually Karina's, and it usually needs charging. Overnight, mine is always by my bed, on charge. Right next to me. If it had taken place in a different room, how much time would have been lost trying to find either phone? Then the phone had to have a signal. Usually, there's no issue with this but sometimes, unexplainably, the signal drops. On this occasion, it didn't.

Karina got onto the phone straight away and kept herself together enough to explain which service she wanted and to explain the situation to the responder on the line. What if the responder hadn't been at her best? What if it had been the end of a long shift and she was knackered or dare I say it, not even especially good at her job? What if the responder had been unable to build that immediate and necessary trust with Karina, that they, the responder had the skills to help, but that she had to listen and follow instructions to the letter?

What if Karina had been so overwhelmed with panic that she couldn't absorb the instructions? What if she had done everything instructed by the responder, but not quite right, not quite hard enough, not quite in the right place? What if Karina couldn't overcome the negative effect of the mattress absorbing the compressions? What if she'd tired to the point of exhaustion and couldn't continue with the CPR?

What if the nearest Paramedics had been just too far away? What if the traffic hadn't moved over quick enough? What if roadworks and temporary lights had slowed down usual response times? What if there had been a traffic accident? What if it had happened an hour or so earlier during the school run? What if all available resources were occupied with other life-threatening scenarios? Or, as is becoming increasingly the case, what if too many ambulances and Paramedics were stuck in a queue outside an A&E?

What if the Paramedics had gone to our neighbour's house first? All too often we get each other's taxis, pizzas, and Amazon deliveries. Karina had to break away from me, run downstairs to open the front door for the Paramedics. What if that had taken longer? If she'd been less fit, or had tripped? (Which she did but didn't fall.)

What if I hadn't responded to the second shock? Would there have been a third? Or a fourth? What if my body had been just a little bit weaker? What if my heart had become damaged during the cardiac arrest?

There were so many links in the chain. So many opportunities for the process *not* to work. The planets had to have lined up perfectly. It would have only taken one of those things to have been slightly out of alignment, only slightly, and the end result we had, couldn't have been reached.

I kept coming back to it: *I'm never that lucky.*

Given there was only one set of circumstances in which a favourable outcome could have been achieved - not one of the above things could have gone wrong - I was beginning to feel an 8% success rate was quite high. It seemed there were so many combinations for any number of the conditions to have not gone my way, that the odds of failure were so much higher than 92%. The upside of this thinking was that I became more resolved than ever, to do more of what I enjoyed in this new life and less of what I didn't. It seemed a reasonable direction of travel, given everything that had happened. But there was also a downside to this reflection on the probabilities and outcomes. Almost inevitably I zoned in on this narrowest of survival windows, trying to work out what it meant to me, to know that once, albeit briefly, my heart had stopped and I wasn't breathing. I was dead.

What if I had stayed dead?

Following my discharge from hospital, there were several dates of significance on the calendar, starting with Fathers' Day. But then over the coming weeks and months, other dates or events of note included George's 18th birthday, getting his first car, his A' Level results and heading off to University in September. There was also Ben's 15th birthday and our Wedding anniversary to celebrate.

All these events took on new levels of significance and appreciation. We were all very aware of how different they would have been, had I not been there. The dates or events would have come and gone whether I was there or not, but they would have been muted by the distraction of my absence. And that made me sad. Very sad for the *imagined* pain of my family and how close it had come to being made real.

Our minds don't have fixed boundaries. Imagination builds cities, relationships, and cures disease. But it can also lead us to all kinds of unhelpful places. Sometimes our minds make us feel like a passenger in our own existence, taking us on a journey not necessarily of our own choosing. The combination of thinking about the slimmest of opportunities for a successful outcome and contemplating what life would be like for my family had I not been revived, kept bringing me back to that question and it was to occupy my mind for some time.

What if I had stayed dead?

What if there was some other parallel Universe in which everything as I know it, still existed, except me? My family continued to live on without me, upset and grieving and incredibly unhappy. They'd have the rest of their lives to live out, but with their husband, dad, brother, uncle no longer physically around. I would gradually fade into a memory; my life with them being slowly distilled down into a collection of memories and stories. Just as happens to everyone who has ever lived.

This was an upsetting thought, but I reasoned with myself that yes, what if that parallel Universe did exist and my family were living in that scenario? It had no bearing on me at all – I no longer existed in that Universe – my consciousness was here, in this one. This was my focus. This was my reality.

But my mind hadn't finished with me. Because then it dawned on me: this may be my reality now, but is this the *real* reality? It's all very well adopting the stance that because I no longer exist in the parallel Universe, then that Universe is relegated to a second-tier; having only pretend or imaginary status. But what if this Universe is the second tier? What if the other, Karl-less Universe is the main one? The real one? What if I'm living in *Plan B*?

Being dead was a significant event in the other Universe and yet here I was. Did I jump track? Am I on a branch line, away from that main track? The numbers were stacked in that direction. There were 92 chances out of 100 that I wouldn't have continued along that original track. Contemplating your existence may not be real, is tantamount to considering whether you're a ghost. And if you are, does anything really matter?

I know what you're thinking - that I was way overthinking this, and you're absolutely right. But sometimes we lose mastery of our thinking and become subservient to it. That's an enduring trait of the human mind. The voice we hear the most, on a daily basis, is our own, in our own mind. For good or bad, there it is, every woken minute, channelling our thoughts. Sometimes it's our biggest champion; far too often it can be our biggest bully and sometimes it cooks up a collection of bizarre, irrational stories or thoughts, then turns around to us and says, *'I'll just leave that one with you then, yeah? Get back to me when you've sorted it out.'*

I did sort it out, eventually. I could have gone to counselling but I wanted to work it through on my own. With hindsight, maybe I should have gone because ultimately, I'd still have to work things through, but a counsellor could have given me the tools to speed up the process of getting this shit out of my head. A bit like a mental laxative.

By September, after thinking about my parallel Universe on loop for far too long, I eventually came to the only conclusion I could live with: this is the only Universe in which I'm aware I exist and therefore it's probably safe, and certainly more productive, to put all my emotional eggs in this basket. I certainly couldn't control anything in any other Universe, so it was probably best just to let my grieving family get on with it in Uni#2. Besides, it also began to dawn on me, why should there just only be *one* other parallel Universe? There may be two. Or ten. Or a million. If you really want to push the concept, there could be an infinite number of parallel Universes to consider.

Whilst contemplating the potential for an infinite number of Universes in which I could be dead, alive or somewhere in between being physically and mentally damaged, I began to realise there had been a reason why I hadn't pursued Quantum Physics as a career. Well, two actually. The first was that I wasn't even bright enough to take Physics as an O' Level, never mind the fantasy version. The second, however, is that I *was* bright enough to appreciate that if you wander around gazing at your navel, at some point you're going to bump into something - and it'll hurt.

My mind was already hurting, trying to wade through all these thoughts. Ultimately, I think I just ran out of available energy to get to any sort of conclusion, so I parked that quantum conundrum. But Gordon had been right on the money when he'd said sometimes my body would be ahead and sometimes my mind.

I'd had a weekend away planned with my brother Mark, as my joint Christmas and Birthday gift to him. I'm like that. I like to save on gift tags by getting just the one combined present. Towards the end of July, we were to hire a fisherman's cottage on the coast near Whitby in a little village called Staithes. The plan was to get there on the Friday, walk along the coast to Whitby on the Saturday and on the Sunday, we were going out on a small fishing boat to catch mackerel and cod and would cook it on the harbourside. Prior to me being hospitalised, we couldn't wait to get going on our adventure, although we'd mentally cancelled it once the bypass had been decided.

There's a difference between mentally cancelling something and *physically* cancelling something. The date of our weekend was ten weeks following my operation. I genuinely hadn't given it much thought during the first half of my recovery, beyond it being off, because, how on earth could it be on? But I hadn't physically cancelled the Airbnb. There was a flexible cancellation option that favoured my preferred stance, which was to wait until one minute to midnight before pulling the plug.

With about four weeks to go, I'd begun to wonder. Everything was progressing well. Mr D had signed me off; Cardiac Rehab was showing weekly improvements and my confidence was returning. *What if...* we still went away but didn't do the fishing trip or the coastal walk. It'd be brilliant to get away for a few days with my Bro. We could potter around the village, have a few pub lunches, do a bit of reading – basically chill out, overlooking a beautiful ancient coastal harbour. Who wouldn't want a slice of that? Besides, I was still in constant need of evidence I was progressing and moving away from Ground Zero. A weekend away with my Bro would be a huge sign that *normality* was returning. I put him on standby, pending further progress reports.

By the end of June, I'd been home for over four weeks. I was doing almost everything for myself but there were still so many elements of support and scaffolding in place. I was no longer Mr Daisy and had moved to the front passenger seat, but nonetheless was still being driven around and wincing as we drove over speed bumps. I was still attending clinics to have my ulcerous wound dressings changed. I was rarely left unattended and my lovely Mother-in-Law, Christine, was still staying at our house, as she had done since two days after my run-in with the Paramedics.

Our family wouldn't have gotten by without her support. She was the glue that helped hold everyone together. As well as the glamour jobs such as washing, ironing, and tidying, she also provided emotional support and company for Karina and the boys – and me, once I'd returned home. I'll be eternally grateful to her and owe her quite a debt. Including introducing me to the guilty pleasure of watching Judge Rinder.

With two weeks to go to the trip and the Airbnb cancellation deadline looming, we decided the weekend was on. We would do as much or as little as we wanted, or rather, as I was capable of. That the weekend was going ahead caused a noticeable disturbance in The Force for Karina. She was quite anxious for my welfare, which was understandable although I was quite dismissive of it at the time. I was feeling stronger and more capable with each day that passed. I'd been for a few local, sunny rural walks with my buddy. They'd been slow, steady strolls, mostly on the flat but between 1½ to 2½ hours which had felt like milestone achievements. We'd even finished them off with a couple of shandies at conveniently placed hostelries.

The ulcer on my chest wound had finally sealed over, was repairing well and I'd even driven myself to the final few appointments to have the dressing changed. Life was beginning to take shape into something I recognised and was enjoying again. With that in mind, it seemed only obvious to me that I would be driving myself to Staithes on the Yorkshire coast, a journey of approximately 145 miles and just under three hours travel.

Karina saw things differently judging by the Vesuvian eruption when I casually dropped this into conversation. I really couldn't see the issue. There had been times when I'd regularly drive four hours each way on the same day, for a business meeting. However, in a move to appease, I softened my proposal to a holding statement of, 'Let's decide nearer the time, but really, it's up to me.' So, not much softer. I just wanted to retain the right to decide.

I could see something was happening though. Karina's response had been seismic; a definite overreaction in my opinion. That said, there had been a gradual shifting of the emotional tectonic plates over the previous weeks. Since the cardiac arrest Karina had been the strong one; delivering CPR, providing physical help and emotional support; protecting me from situations and to some extent from myself if I appeared to be overdoing something. She had been the leader, the one in front taking the headwind on my behalf whilst all the while reaching backwards with her hand out for me to hold on to. She had been my guide, pulling me along the road to recovery.

And she had done a wonderfully astounding job of it because there I was, with a weekend away with my Bro on the horizon. But you can't take on that role and fulfil that sort of responsibility unless you're incredibly strong. Strong physically, mentally, and emotionally – all of which can be very draining and tiring.

In the weeks preceding, I was clearly making considerable progress, certainly physically. Mentally too in the sense of being more confident and having an ever-increasing belief that my recovery wouldn't suddenly reverse for whatever reason. Sure, at that time, I was still very much in the existential dogfight of contemplating the parallel Universe in which I didn't exist. But apart from not being 100% sure I was still operating in my core life and the world I saw and felt was genuinely real, mentally I was in good shape.

The progress I'd been making meant I was relying on Karina less and less. And if I were to truly recover, this was always going to happen. It had to, otherwise, I couldn't honestly claim to be recovering, or at some point, to have finally recovered. I had no idea where that finish line was or what the criteria were to say I'd crossed the line, but ultimately, it was my goal. It was still some way off, but my progress overall had been considerable. Modesty prevents me from using the word *exponential* but if I'd been told when in ICU that I'd be on a weekend away with my Bro within 9 weeks or so, I'd have assumed that the grasshoppers had taken over the asylum.

By mid-July, most aspects of my emotional and physical reliance on Karina for recovery had all but disappeared. This was becoming apparent by the nature of the conversations relating to my weekend away. It was beginning to feel that in some aspects of my recovery, I'd moved ahead of Karina. That I was pulling away with the willingness to challenge myself more; to seek the enjoyment of the outdoor life I'd craved and set as a goal, back in the days when I was creeping my fingers up the wall to stretch frozen muscles. I enjoyed this sense of progress and being able to expand and test my capabilities. I only saw an upside.

Karina has always been more risk-averse than I and clearly had concerns about the weekend. Especially the notion of me driving there and back, given I hadn't driven any great distance since mid-April. I could see it was worrying her and that she was carrying this worry around almost all the time. It dawned on me that this wasn't fair. It wasn't fair that after all this time and all the energy my wife had put into caring for me; supporting and protecting me; that just when I was feeling the best I'd felt for months (which of course is where she wanted me to be), she was feeling a bit shit and a bit left behind. And it was more than a bit my fault. I took myself off to one side for a little conversation and thought about things from her point of view. On reflection, and it really didn't take me that long, I realised the idea of me driving wasn't the best one I'd had that year. In fact, it was pretty stupid. I probably could have done it at a push, but I'd have been knackered and would have hated it. Then I'd have been really pissed off with myself for realising that Karina had been right, I'd been wrong, and I'd still have the drive back to contend with. Double pisser.

So, it was agreed, I'd get the train to York, where Mark would meet me and he'd drive us to the coast, via a lunch stop in Pickering. That, as it turned out, was a fantastically enjoyable journey, one which I'd never swap. Karina was good with this arrangement too. She still had her concerns for the weekend, but more so just because it was my first true release back into the wild, albeit with my big Bro to keep an eye on me. I realised, or perhaps was reminded at that point, it was all very well being ahead in some aspects of my recovery but having been pulled along by Karina for so long, on some occasions, it was now my role to turn around and reach out a hand to her, to help pull her along with me. We'd both been through a lot, and we were both on this journey together. In my race to recover, I'd lost sight of that a little. That said, I'd felt like I'd been so needy for so long, that to feel needed again, even just a little bit, felt quite good.

The weekend itself was bloody brilliant! We explored the village, had those pub lunches and slipped into the slow life. We went out on the boat, caught our mackerel, and chatted with the fisherman and his wife as we prepared our evening meal on the harbourside. Everything was just as we'd originally planned and hoped. I'd taken my walking boots *just in case* and on the Saturday, we set off on a little cliff top saunter along The Cleveland Way. A leisurely bimble which yes, did also include a pub lunch. It was mostly sunny, and we talked and walked and walked and talked. Unbelievably we'd covered ten miles by the time we stopped. (We got the bus back.) Ten miles is a decent walk anyway, but ten weeks after a cardiac arrest and open-heart surgery – I was genuinely staggered, but most definitely not staggering. I was on a massive high and it felt like the endpoint of the first stage of my recovery.

The next stages would be re-engaging with work-life and working out what my future, second life would be about. What I had worked out though, was that this sort of thing had to be a part of it. Creating the time and space to relax and enjoy life rather than constantly forging the resilience to grind through work. It sounds a cliché but there's always some truth in them. Work had mostly been my life, so there'd been little balance. But as I'd seen the other side - or not, as the case may be - that would have to change. I'll always remember that weekend with my big Bro. It was only the cliff tops we'd climbed and walked but for me, it felt like I'd conquered Everest.

# 30

# Can I Have A Word?

*"Courage doesn't always roar.*
*Sometimes courage is the quiet voice at the end of the day saying:*
*'I will try again tomorrow'."*
**Mary Anne Radmacher**

Although I'd already decided that when I did go back to work, full time for me, would be three days a week, I'd done nothing about making it a reality. I still had to reconnect with my business so from mid-August, had a series of meetings with my deputy, our Account Director, in a Starbucks at a nearby hotel. We had a meeting room at the office, but at that stage, I really wasn't up for a whole string of, 'How are you?' conversations. I had to start wrapping my head around the status of the business, but the meetings also gave me the chance to see where she was up to with the MBO. Exiting the business would dovetail perfectly with the notion of the second life I was so keen to craft.

The long and short of it was, they'd been so busy on all the client projects that nothing much had happened on the MBO. I shouldn't have been surprised. The team would've been up against it had I been there, so were even more so, during my absence. Even so, the lack of progress was a great disappointment for me. I'd wanted *out* the year before, hence me initiating the conversation. I knew an exit would take a while but was beginning to wonder if it would happen via this route. I kept this disappointment to myself though, grateful for my deputy holding the fort during my forced leave.

We discussed current client projects; how events that I'd missed, had gone; business development and of course HR. The whole team had done an amazing job under challenging circumstances. Clients were happy and we had new business leads in the pipeline. My deputy was brilliant during these meetings. I could tell there'd been a few staff and project challenges, but she didn't burden me with them. There'd be some sort of reveal further down the line but just as she was happy to hold back, I was happy not to dig. As I later discovered, the challenges weren't unmanageable but even just knowing they existed, piqued my early warning system, and reinforced my desire to exit the business.

I have to say though, my deputy had done an amazing job, in what had been our busiest time, in what ended up being the best financial year in our history. She'd protected me from the business and had barely contacted me except to see how I was getting on. I doubt my mental recovery would have gone as well as it had if I'd thrown myself back into work mode earlier. She'd ensured I hadn't even needed to dip my toe into work waters and Karina and I were hugely grateful for that. I told her so at the first meeting and when I think of all the people who, combined, were involved in getting me fixed and back on my feet, I will always include her.

I had a further two meetings throughout August and we arranged a date for my first day back in the office. I'd asked for no fuss to be made, which of course they all completely ignored. There were *Welcome Back* banners around the place, my desk had cards and chocolates piled up and the office dog (hers actually) wouldn't leave me alone – which was all rather lovely.

I did one day the first week, two the following and then three the week after that. But that third week, we were running an event in Leicester, which I desperately wanted to attend because 1) I'd worked on it for almost 18 months before I went off sick and 2) Brian Cox was one of the speakers and I wasn't going to let that selfie opportunity pass me by.

I only allowed myself very light duties and it was fantastic to be in the thick of an event again, albeit mostly as a spectator. I had to buy myself a new suit though. Although I'd put weight back on during my recovery, I was still probably a stone lighter than the last event I'd attended in April. At least I felt I looked the part of an MD, even if I didn't do an awful lot on the event. I got my selfie with Brian Cox too. Writing this prompted me to dig that photo out of my phone and I was quite shocked at how gaunt and old I had looked, despite how positive I felt about myself at the time. Another reminder of the power of perspective.

Over the coming weeks, I didn't get too involved with the projects we were handling. Everyone already had their allocated roles and was getting on with them. I occasionally acted as a sounding board but was pretty much left alone. I was beginning to wonder how I was going to contribute to the company, such was my level of project detachment. As every business owner knows though, there are no end of *House* projects and it was those that I began to get stuck into. I spent most of the rest of the year, working on the website, updating, slightly redesigning, modifying the Search Engine Optimisation along with forecasting and planning for 2020.

However, around the middle of October, my workload increased significantly. The 2020 projects were well into the planning stages, and I began to pick up various tasks. I also had to initiate activity I really didn't enjoy but was unquestionably my responsibility: recruitment. Recruitment can be for positive or negative reasons –

expansion or replacement. Initially, we needed to quickly search for a new Office Manager as ours had resigned due to her relocating.

My deputy was also involved in the process, especially during the interview stage, but the preliminary work - creating and posting the ads, revising job descriptions, sifting CVs - was mine. I used to say, '*You only had to be good to be better than most,*' when looking at CVs. My God. I honestly didn't know how unemployment was so low. As I waded through the applications, I knew it wasn't going to be a quick fix as, by then, it appeared, '*You only had to be shit to be better than most.*' People were either incapable of reading the requirements of the ad or checking their own applications. But mostly, it seemed, both.

We'd also identified the need for another Account Manager so had started recruitment for that role, in addition to wanting to offer work experience to four, 3rd-year Event Management students – yet more recruitment. That we were taking on rather than replacing, was a positive thing. Unfortunately, however, the process is still the same: a painful journey wading through applications from people, some of whom, were either so ill-suited to the job descriptions or blatantly apathetic in their applications. Tits on a fish would've been more use. Then there were others whose applications suggested a very unique interpretation to the phrase *attention to detail*. Remembering to flush may have pushed their boundaries. Recruitment is a time consuming and mostly fruitless journey. Trying to fill these six roles was taking up increasing amounts of my day-to-day life.

At the end of October, my recruitment burden was compounded when one of our Account Executives handed in her notice, to take a role in North Wales, nearer to where she lived. Whilst I could understand her motives, this meant yet more of my time was spent sifting applications from self-entitled folk who seemed to think their Instagram accounts alone should be enough to get them a job.

By mid-November, I was juggling the update of the website, 2020 project planning and recruitment for seven roles, including sifting and carrying out first and second interviews. Collectively, this wasn't conducive to a three-day week, which is why I found myself working five days as standard, to work around candidate availability for interviews.

By the beginning of December, after the most intensive recruitment phase I could recall, we'd managed to appoint the Office Manager, the Account Executive, and the four student work experience roles, leaving only the Account Manager role unfilled. We had a raft of second interviews lined up though, so things were looking up.

That said, the whole process had left me feeling jaded and off-beam with the way I'd envisaged my new role and life panning out. There'd also been very little movement on the MBO apart from the 2020 forecasts being updated. By then, we'd been talking for almost 18 months. In all honesty, I was beginning to regret not having gone out to the market for the sale. I bore my deputy no bad feeling about this, but as time went on, I sensed a fear in her about the *risk* of taking the business on. There are no guarantees in business. That's the nature of being an entrepreneur. You accept some level of risk but then get to take the gains. I was feeling frustrated, tired, but above all, disappointed that my vision of a more balanced life had become a blur in such a short space of time. But still, Christmas was around the corner.

Christmas was always a big thing at Assured Events. Legendary even. Everyone received chocolate advent calendars on 1st December and *Tree Up Day* was in our diaries before the last of the summer sunscreen had been shelved. The day of our Christmas *do* would start with me having arranged for everyone to have their preferred breakfast waiting for them as they arrived at the office. This would be followed by fizz, Secret Santa and a Christmas Quiz I'd prepared with prizes and gifts from the company. Over the years, the quiz had taken on a life all of its own. Some staff even revised Christmas TV ads, in case they came up! It's fair to say, they were a competitive bunch.

After a few hours, we'd jump into taxis, head to the airport, and fly off somewhere for an overnight stay. Always somewhere Christmassy and ideally, somewhere cold, and snowy. That year it was Oslo. We'd crawl the bars, have a meal, hit a club or late bar, and have more laughs than we could remember. It was always a slow start the following day and we'd be back at Manchester airport by about 6pm. The company paid for everything, and the staff had two days off at no cost to their annual leave allowance. It was my way of saying *thank you* at the end of each year. (But just to be clear, I did say thank you to them more than once a year!) The team loved our Christmas dos. So did I. Who wouldn't?

I know putting on a Christmas like this made even more work for me, but I loved giving our team something back, the laughs we had and the stories we came back with. And stories there were. Each trip generated its own raft of tales, mishaps, and mayhem. I hope they'll all remember those Assured Events Christmases as being the best of their work lives.

At the end of the first day back in the office after we returned from Oslo, one of the Account Executives asked if they could *have a word*. *Having a word* was never a good sign. Nobody ever asks the MD for *a word* to tell them what a great job they're doing and how appreciated they are.

It transpired that, during the return journey from Oslo, she had accepted a job offer and was handing in her one-month notice. I was incredibly disappointed she'd accepted a job offer whilst returning from our fully expensed Christmas jolly. But more than that, I was being given very little opportunity to get any traction on recruitment, as we'd be shutting down for the best part of two weeks in a matter of days. This generated a fair bit of upset and anxiety in me, knowing I had to jump back into recruitment firefighting, in addition to still trying to fill the other outstanding role.

People leave. I get it. It's what people do. That's business. But timing and how I was already feeling about my trashed vision of a more balanced life, amplified the impact.

Whenever people left the company, I was always aware of how much it destabilised others in the team – and understandably so. Not only would the remaining team members be losing a reliable teammate and possibly a genuine mate, but they also had to learn to trust a new person. An unknown person with an unknown skill set and unknown levels of reliability. And of course, there was never any chance of the new person being in place before the old one left. All of which would inevitably mean more workload temporarily coming the way of the remaining team members. I was obliged to tell my deputy about the resignation but decided to wait until January to tell the team. There was no point in souring their Christmases with work worries.

I was being pulled away from the second life I'd envisaged. If at its simplest level, I'd wanted my new life to be filled with more things I enjoyed and less of what I didn't, then I was going backwards. My life was seemingly filling up with the stuff I didn't enjoy and was choking anything I did enjoy. It saddened me to feel my hopes for the life I'd imagined were sliding away, after only such a short time of re-engaging with the company. The company I'd created.

A week later and just days before we broke for Christmas, one of our Senior Account Managers asked if she could *have a quick word* at the end of the day. My heart sank. I already knew what was coming. As we sat down in the meeting room, she was already glassy-eyed. '*There's no easy way to say this...*'

She was resigning and giving me her three-month notice. She had a young family and was commuting over an hour each way, following a relatively recent relocation. Again, I got it. I understood her reasoning and couldn't argue against it. But from my perspective, she'd been with us for 8½ years, she was great at her job, and it felt like having an arm ripped off at the worst possible time. I wanted to vomit at the thought of the mountain to climb in terms of recruitment but more significantly, the level of experience we were losing. She kindly offered to work beyond her three months as she had no role to go to, which I was genuinely grateful for. But then I did wonder why I was being told just before the break. Once again, I had no opportunity of starting any meaningful recruitment process beyond posting the ads and then having it weigh heavily on me over the festive period. And once again, I had to tell my deputy but needless to say, this news was also kept from the team so they could enjoy their Christmases protected from the worry of the inevitable turmoil that lay ahead.

Looking through the lens of the new life that I'd vowed to create having survived my cardiac arrest and heart bypass, I had an overwhelming sense of being cheated with no means of appeal. I was struggling to see how I could reverse the situation. I was being dragged by a current of my own making, further and further away from the safety of a balanced and rewarding life. There was also a part of me that was envious, or possibly even resentful, that others could just walk away. I couldn't. It's worth pointing out, we didn't usually have this level of churn. Most of the team had been with us for many years. It almost felt as if the moves had been held back until my return, which added to my resentment.

That last week was my tipping point. As founder and MD, I had no contract and no one to hand in my notice to. I'd created my own personal Hotel California and I couldn't take much more of it. The

MBO was stalling and the business I'd created was becoming toxic to me. I'm not sure if that's too strong a word, but I don't think so. It's absolutely no reflection on the team who were hard-working, talented, decent people and despite how I felt, as an Agency, we were still delivering fantastic work and were winning new clients. In previous years I would've had the armour to deal with such short-term setbacks and would've had no issues in seeing the bigger, longer-term, successful picture. The issue was me. I simply no longer had the resilience or was the right person for the role of leading the business.

I recognised I may have to forget the sale and drop the idea of the MBO being my ticket out. The possibility of a nuclear option still existed. Closing Assured Events and just walking away was beginning to look like my only route to getting anywhere close to being able to enjoy the second life I'd been given. I resolved to give this some serious thought over the Christmas break. In the meantime, I had the pressing issue of having to drive to a Services on the M62 to collect my Mum from my brother as she was staying with us for ten days over Christmas. So, it was with a heavy heart I set off to pick her up but told myself I couldn't allow how I was feeling, to affect her stay. She deserved to have a lovely Christmas and seeing her son, miserable and trapped wouldn't deliver her that. So, I rallied, buried my feelings, and put on my game face.

Ho! Ho! Ho!

# 31

## So This Is Christmas

*"Happiness is not the absence of problems.*
*It's the ability to deal with them."*
**Steve Maraboli**

For as long as I can remember, the arrangement had been that Mum alternated her Christmases between Mark and me. It probably started a few years after Dad had died and coincided with Karina and I getting married a few years later. Mum loved it, we loved having her and it also gave my brother a break from being the *son-on-call*, as he lived just a few miles from Mum.

Mum was 87 and until the last few years, had been quite robust. I mean she had a stack of health issues, but she was a tough old bird. Until a couple of years prior, if you ignored the fact her medical records were always wheeled in on their own dedicated trolley, you'd have said that she was in pretty good shape.

By then, however, she was on $O^2$ permanently and had been for a couple of years. There was an oxygen machine at her house which sounded like Darth Vader snoozing and if she ever went out anywhere, she was accompanied by an $O^2$ travel cylinder. So, in readiness for her stay, we'd had an oxygen machine delivered along with a stack of travel cylinders. She could cover very short distances with the assistance of a walking stick but really, a wheelchair was needed for anywhere outside of the house, so had hired one of those too.

It must have been difficult for Mum to see this decline in herself. Our parents had once been part of a World Champion Formation Dancing team in the 50s and 60s. They'd travelled to competitions in Europe and had appeared on TV dozens of times. In middle age, they'd opened a dance school and were Kevin and Joanne Clifton's first ballroom dancing teachers when they were kids. Dancing had been Mum & Dad's passion and gliding around a ballroom was as easy and obvious to them as walking is to everyone else. So, accepting such poor levels of mobility now was exceptionally challenging.

I'd only seen Mum in October a couple of months before, so I was quite shocked when I arrived at the Services and saw how much she'd deteriorated. Her posture had aged. Her movements were lacking confidence; her strength had been sapped; but more than all of that, she seemed to have retreated into herself. Mum had always been chatty, but much less so now. She was talking certainly, but not very much. She was becoming a recluse in her own frail body.

That said, she was still very excited to be at ours for Christmas and was looking forward to seeing Karina and the boys. The boys always called her *Seaside*, as in Seaside Grandma because she lived near the sea, which she loved. Much fuss was made of her when she arrived, and we put the bag loads of gifts she'd brought around the tree. Once mum was settled down in her chair in front of the log burner and TV, that was it. She was asleep before I could put the kettle on. This was going to be a low maintenance ten days, I thought.

How those next ten days unfolded couldn't have been further from that thought.

Mum had a little fall the following day, which required an emergency Doctor prescribing pain killers. Although tailing off towards the end of the visit, that pain stayed with Mum the whole time. Getting in and out of bed was a problem. Getting to the bathroom was a problem. She went off her food. Her sleeping was awful as she couldn't lay down due to the pain, so started sleeping in an armchair. If I'd been shocked at how much Mum had deteriorated when I'd picked her up, she'd gone downhill since she'd been with us. Exponentially downhill.

It was heart-breaking. Truly heart-breaking.

Within 24 hours, Karina and I had become full-time carers. I'd gone into Christmas desperately needing some breathing space; feeling choked with work and full of resentment at being unable to enjoy the chance of the second life I'd been given. And now this. There was no air pocket. The demands of delivering Christmas can be tough on their own but unexpectedly being appointed as a full-time carer whilst trying to manage my own emotional state - I felt robbed and stretched thinner than ever.

It was as if I had no control over anything. I was seemingly at the behest of the Universe pushing me around however it wanted, and I couldn't do a single thing about it. I was in a nosedive I couldn't pull out of. It's a herculean task to try and keep perspective when you feel like that. I tried to apply the Shitometer to the situation, whereby 10 is *I'm already dead* so maybe 9 is life-threatening. I'm not sure what words should be attributed to 8 but this felt like an 8. Some days it felt like a 9 because my second life was totally threatened. The aim of the scale is to apply perspective; to turn the dial down and recognise that really, it's not an 8, it's a 4, maybe a 5. But I couldn't. Because I was constantly on call. And after the Christmas break, I knew I'd be straight back into constantly being on call fighting fires at work.

Don't get me wrong, there are some good memories of that time too. We got Mum out to the Park in the wheelchair and took her to Jus and Sarah's on Boxing Day. We had some lovely chats too. But the anxiety created by the intensity of the caring and knowing what

I was walking back into at work, never left me. One or the other would have been just about manageable and bearable. But the two compounded each other.

I only had it for ten days. How do people cope when that's their entire life? Day in day out. Those people are living, breathing Saints. And thinking about that made me feel shallow and pathetic and self-ish. And at that moment in time, I think I was all those things. I didn't want to be, but I was.

I was at a loss as to why I'd been spared those months earlier. Nothing was different in my life. If anything, it was worse. I was still the buffer taking the pounding. I was absorbing all the shit which seemed to originate far away from me but none the less, gravitate to-wards me.

By the time I took Mum back to hand over to Mark, she'd be-come a shell of the person she'd been when I'd collected her. And she'd already become a shadow at that point. My Bro was visibly shocked when he saw her. He was also distressed at the realisation that the role of full-time carer was being transferred to him, at least in the short term, as Mum was clearly unable to live on her own, un-aided. We also knew we were already well past the point of looking into sheltered accommodation. It felt like the only option was the nuclear one. The one Mum had always dreaded and had said she never wanted to fall back on – a care home. But how long would that take to arrange? Neither of us had any idea but could guess there wasn't a switch somewhere which would see it sorted by teatime. During the journey back to the east coast, my brother said Mum only mumbled two words and one of those was in her sleep.

After he pulled away from the car park at the Services, I realised I wasn't in the best of shape. I had over an hour of motorway driving ahead of me and wasn't really in the frame of mind, so stayed a while in the hope the mood would pass. I was considering going back in to get another coffee when I suddenly had an overwhelming sense that I'd seen my Mum for the last time. I sat there for about 20 minutes, numb, unravelling, oblivious to people walking past. I was also oblivious to the ANPR cameras clocking I'd overstayed the two-hour limit on free parking and was already in the process of receiving a £120 parking fine.

Some days you're the pigeon and others you're the statue.

# 32

## Stuck In Reverse

*"You, me, or nobody is gonna hit as hard as life. But it ain't how hard you can hit. It's about how hard you can get hit, and keep moving forwards."*
**Rocky Balboa**

I couldn't shake the thought I'd seen my Mum for the last time, so early the next morning Karina and I drove over to Cleethorpes. Regardless of my state of mind, the way events had unfolded overnight meant we would have made the journey anyway. Mum had said very little since she'd got back home. She'd also eaten and drunk very little. By morning an ambulance had been called and Mum had been taken to hospital.

She was on a standard ward but looked dreadful. Terribly emaciated, ashen, her eyes sunken, carrying heavy lilac bags. Mum had never been tall; she would have claimed 5ft 1 at the height of her dancing powers. But over recent years, she'd retreated closer to the ground she'd shuffled across. But there, lying in that hospital bed, she looked even tinier, barely taking up space under the covers.

We'd asked a Doctor for an update, and he took us all into an unoccupied side room. Never a good sign. Their initial concern had been regarding Sepsis but this had proved unfounded. Nonetheless, Mum appeared to have an infection somewhere. The Doctor was exceptionally gifted in that rarest of skills; the one where both good and bad news are delivered simultaneously without generating the joy or pain usually attributed to either. It's the medical equivalent of attempting a controlled explosion. He was confident that for now, Mum was ok but that ultimately, he'd be surprised if she made it through this. It seemed that Mum was well beyond the tipping point.

There were no concessions and we left at 8pm, albeit fully expecting a phone call before we were next allowed on the ward the following day at 2pm. No such call was received and our morning call was slightly surprising in that she'd had a good night; had enjoyed some breakfast and was feeling much brighter. This wasn't the news we were expecting but understandably, were over the moon about.

We were astounded by the difference in the person we'd left only the evening before. Mum was chatty, lucid, and completely engaging with us. Don't get me wrong; she wasn't going to be leaving there any day soon, but the transformation was miraculous. As an atheist, not a word I would ever really use.

The Universe had given us a massive win.

Mum remained in hospital for just over two weeks. During this time, we managed to find some regular care support to visit her throughout the day, for when she was back at home.

After being discharged, Mum was only at home for a few days but was then readmitted in pretty much the same condition as when she'd previously gone into hospital. Once again, we found ourselves in discussions with an overworked A&E Doctor. Whilst he'd liked to have seen higher functionality across the board, he was adamant that at that point in time, she was very stable. As such we decided to head back to Manchester. We all said our goodbyes but I couldn't help but have a sense of déjà vu.

I'd kept in touch with Mark throughout the following day but to my surprise, just as I was leaving work at about 6pm I got a call from Mum. She was very distraught and wanted me to tell Mark to go and collect her. She claimed people weren't being very nice to her. It was difficult to maintain a conversation as her thread was incoherent. I suspected her kidney infection was at the root of this confusion, but it was still distressing to hear. She sounded so frightened. I phoned Mark who said he'd call her but was going to visit that evening anyway.

As I pulled up at the gym, I phoned Mum to let her know that my Bro was going in to visit her and her relief was palpable. As was mine. There's something hard about being the child yet having to console a parent.

Whilst still in the gym at about 8:10pm, I could see Mark was phoning me. I cut short my session and took the call whilst heading to my car. He told me Mum had calmed down and she knew she was being a bit irrational. She'd also accepted that hospital was where she needed to be. She was much more content and relaxed as well as appreciative of Mark going in to visit again. He'd also been told by nurses that Mum's numbers were stable and there was nothing to be overly concerned about. I was so relieved that this episode had resolved itself. It had been awful hearing Mum so afraid and upset.

When I got home at 8:30pm, I was bringing Karina up to speed on developments, when the hospital phoned me. A nurse introduced herself and explained she was going through Mum's file and noticed there were two numbers for her sons. She asked if I was the son who'd just visited, and I explained that had been my brother as I lived in Manchester. Her tone was very light, and matter of fact and she apologised for the confusion in their records and said she'd update them. She then went on to say that she hoped I would be able to appreciate the importance of her knowing exactly who she's talking to, as she was sorry to have to tell me that, 'Your Mum has just passed.'

Nothing can prepare you for those words. There were only five of them but getting my head around them caused so much confusion. I appreciate the word *passed* is often used to deliver news of death. It's more for the teller than the receiver. For them, it feels less harsh and lessens the blow they're delivering, which is: someone has died. Stopped living. Is no more. Saying someone has *died* is more finite, colder, less empathetic perhaps. But it's all semantics. The result is the same. I'd have preferred the word *died* because, although it only takes a fraction of a second, the brain still has to go through the process of translating the word *passed* to *that's it – game over – forever*. No Court of Appeal. No opportunity to say or do anything else. No one to moan to or to try and get the decision overturned. Time's up.

If you're prepared for it, if you're expecting it, the translation time is barely perceptible because, well, you're expecting it and your receptors are ready to pick up any such linguistic nuances. But when you're unprepared for it, it just adds to your initial confusion.

After everything I've detailed running up to this news, it'd be easy to wonder why I felt any degree of confusion at all. But sometimes the context in which we hear the words adds to this confusion, which in my case, was definitely the biggest cause for confusion, for three reasons.

The first was that I'd only spoken to Mum less than two hours before. She hadn't been brilliant, but she'd phoned me; she'd been clear, and she'd been grateful for the news that Mark was visiting again that evening. There's always going to be the last conversation with someone but it's the proximity of it to the time they die that seems to shock us so much. But then, if talking to someone very soon before they died was some kind of measure of how likely it would be for them to die, then hardly anyone would die.

Much more significantly though was that I'd only got off the phone to Mark 15 minutes earlier telling me Mum was in an OK place and the nurses were happy with her numbers and observations. Which not unreasonably, we'd translated into *nothing to immediately worry about*.

But the single biggest aspect of my lack of preparedness was who was giving me the news. Bar the holiday periods during Uni, I've lived away from my hometown all my life. Ever since Mark had phoned to tell me that Dad had died in 1995, I always knew, unless I was there with Mum myself, that 100%, at some point, he'd eventually phone me with this news. For the past, God knows how many years, every time I saw him calling or I'd missed a call, a tiny, little part of me couldn't help but wonder if this was *The Call*. He was even recorded on Mum's medical notes as the first point of contact as next of kin, being only down the road from Mum. I never did find out why I was contacted first. That I was, and it wasn't Mark breaking the news to me had caught me with my guard down. That and the nurse's very neutral and light tone leading up to delivering those five words.

So, despite everything that had been going on with Mum, I was about as unprepared as I could have been, to be told that I was now an orphan. A 51-year-old orphan, granted, but the sense of loss that comes with a second parent dying also translates into a sense of being alone, regardless of what level of support you have from family and friends. Dry January ended that evening.

We drove to Cleethorpes the following morning, met with Mark and his family, and started the two to three weeks of funeral planning and stage one of looking through belongings and paperwork. I wasn't in Cleethorpes that whole time. Initially, it was for about a week and then back and forth. My brother and I were making the arrangements together and there was something comforting in that. Something right. But I was also aware my Assured Events team were under a great deal of strain. Me being away at that time not only compounded the problem in terms of depleted projected handlers, it also meant seeking our recruitment solutions had slowed to a trickle. My deputy could only do so much given the workload she and the team were under. As per usual though, she completely respected where I was at, so hadn't contacted me at all regarding work matters. It's true what they say: times of crises don't build character; they reveal it, and she and the entire Assured Events team, were real stars.

It was all bearing down on me though. My world was stuck firmly in reverse.

I went through many feelings and emotions during that time; the usual range of pain of loss and the anger of grief, all the way to occasional hysteria over stuff that mystified others. One of my more unusual recurring thoughts was how grateful I was I hadn't been one of the 92% for Mum's sake. Well, in this Universe at least. How much it would have hit her, to have to cremate her youngest son. I have no idea why I even gave these wispy thoughts the oxygen to get going. I had enough to contend within the real world without musing over hypothetical reactions to hypothetical events – events that never were. Well, as I kept reminding myself, not in Uni#1, at least.

It was during this early stage of planning for the funeral that we became vaguely aware of a virus outbreak being mentioned in a far-off place called Wuhan, China. None of us had heard of it (Wuhan, that is. China we were vaguely familiar with). There was media talk of the Chinese authorities having to lockdown 10 million citizens in one city. It was one of those stories relating to a part of the world that had no bearing on our lives except as a curious conversation piece.

*How would you go about locking down 10 million people? Only in an authoritarian state like China, would people have no choice but to do as they were told. You wouldn't get that sort of compliance here or in any other democratically run country.*

But in truth, we didn't really give it too much airtime amongst ourselves. We had other things on our minds.

It was comforting when we read the cause of death on Mum's Death Certificate as *frailty of old age*. Basically, her body had run out of energy and had nothing left to give. If I could make it to 87 and have those words on my Death Certificate, I'd regard that as an achievement. The average age of death for a woman in the UK is currently just over 80 years, so Mum topped out at almost 10% over the average, which really is incredible given her list of ailments. So, if ever the term *good innings* applied, I suppose Mum's age would qualify. But for all the truth in the sentiment behind that all too familiar phrase, it doesn't really matter if she'd been 67, 87 or 107... she was my Mum and I missed her terribly.

# 33

# Four Days

*"Here is a test to find out if your mission on Earth is finished.*
*If you're alive, it isn't."*
**Richard Bach**

Mum's packed funeral was on Tuesday 11th February in Grimsby and although I didn't go into the office that week, I was working from home on the Thursday and Friday. There was so much ground to make up on the recruitment drive, I spent those two days sifting through CVs and arranging interviews. We were, by then, desperate for additional support and I knew we were in danger of making the ultimate recruitment mistake. The process was beginning to feel out of control. We needed to take people on to help manage our clients' projects but the urgency for that resource meant we were almost at the point where anyone would do. I was determined to avoid this trap and having to repent down the line.

Finding appropriate CVs was the initial challenge followed by those candidates interviewing well. We were consistently disappointed with the poor level of research candidates had carried out on us. You'd think this would be a basic part of the prep for an interview but sadly very few appeared bothered enough to look beyond the home page of our site. When someone *had* interviewed well, we'd get excited and quickly arrange a second interview. Sometimes these people would then, just not turn up. It's called *ghosting;* abandoning all communication without any explanation, but in truth that's just modern shorthand for being a shit human being. It's fair to say it was a seller's market.

In addition to the increasingly desperate and unproductive recruitment drive and being in the latter stages of preparation for the busiest five-month phase of our year; we were also preparing 2021-23 Project Management Fees for a group of our largest clients. In essence, over the coming weeks, we were pitching for the projects we were currently up to our eyes in, for the next three years. There was no comfy chair.

Meanwhile, the MBO conversation was still live, even if not progressing. *Stalled* was probably the most positive description. I was desperately frustrated but in no position to hassle my deputy. I knew current client projects and the recruitment drive were taking up so much of her time. Showing anything other than gratitude and support would have been grossly unfair. That said, the combined pressure of managing team stresses, recruitment, client projects and pitching were coming together as a Perfect Storm, screaming at me to get out of the business. I was struggling to find any measure of enjoyment in my role or Assured Events. The dream of a three-day week was long gone. I was working long hours across five days and at the weekends. I hadn't even begun to grieve about Mum. I was barely thinking about her given everything going on, which made me feel all the worse whenever she did come into my thoughts. I was stuck in a guilty fog as well as having to manage my own resentment at naively pursuing a single exit strategy. The responsibility for that error of judgement lay entirely with me. I just wanted it all to stop.

By February the World had been introduced to a new term: *Covid-19.* The virus had reached Europe and parts of Italy and Spain were beginning to suffer badly. People were being hospitalised, many were dying, particularly older people and large parts of these countries were being locked down, in much the same way China had done. There were just a handful of cases in the UK, mainly linked to people returning from Wuhan.

By the end of the month, I was very much of the opinion that whilst this was a terrible virus and what was happening to people who were suffering from it was awful, it was effectively a severe flu virus. On 28th February, we had our first inbound enquiry as to whether an event we were running over the week of 28th March, would still be going ahead. That anyone would even consider the event would be cancelled, was greeted with more than a degree of incredulity, by agency and client teams, alike.

On 29th February, there were 23 confirmed cases of Covid-19 in the UK. Some flu seasons cause over 20,000 deaths in the UK. The numbers were incomparable, hence the Cheltenham Festival still went ahead along with European football fixtures. There was even a feeling the media were hyping it up; trying to fill the headline vacuum left by Brexit no longer grabbing the level of attention it previously had.

The following week saw a further 16 enquiries asking the same question about that and other events. Clearly, there was a groundswell of concern, but it was still only averaging just over three enquiries a day. Hardly a tsunami. We'd also had a handful of client conference calls regarding additional measures to minimise the risk of infection and transmission at the events. Scenario modelling was looking at the financial impact, should some attendees pull out. Preparation time was getting short, and the team and I were increasingly frustrated at having to divert so much effort away from urgent project matters and into dealing with these enquiries and initiating additional measures.

By Friday 6$^{th}$ March, concerns regarding the impact of Covid-19 on our events were looking manageable. So much so, that by that date, we'd pressed ahead and filled three of our four vacant positions. One had already started and two had accepted our offers – one on that very day. Things were beginning to look more positive, at least on the recruitment front.

The following week, we received more than 50 enquiries as to whether events were going ahead and clients wanted financial exposure projections, should they postpone or cancel their events. This was new territory for us. All our time and energy was focused on managing the potential impact of Covid-19. In the space of a few days, I'd gone from spinning multiple plates to spinning one: the *what-ifs* caused by Covid-19. Only then was I slapped with the brutal realisation, that what I and many clients had thought was an overhyped flu, was about to hit us hard.

On 11$^{th}$ March, the World Health Organisation declared Covid-19 a global pandemic. Everything unravelled at such a rate of knots, right in front of my eyes: the events; the MBO and the business itself. Within four days, we'd been instructed by all clients to cancel all our events for the rest of the year. There were a couple lined up for the end of the year, but the planning had barely begun and those were put on hold.

We had a team meeting on 17$^{th}$ March, which had been planned for quite a while. Branded and personalised items had been created for everyone and my deputy and I were due to introduce a whole range of measures and incentives, including the new staffing structure. We'd arranged for lunch and gave everyone their personalised items but held back on the plans – they were no longer relevant. Just prior to the meeting, my deputy took me aside and with misty eyes told me she was expecting her second child and wouldn't be pursuing the MBO. I wasn't disappointed or surprised or even angry or upset. Regardless of her pregnancy, I knew I'd missed the boat on the sale of Assured Events. I knew that from there on in, there would be nothing for anyone to buy.

I sent the whole team home after the meeting, to work remotely for the foreseeable future. As they were all packing up their laptops, taking their screens and grabbing boxes of files, one of them said, 'God – I wonder when we'll be back in?'

I already knew, with the same kind of certainty I'd had when the word *pacemaker* was first mentioned; despite me wanting to resist the thought of it, that they'd never be back in. Within the space of a week, Assured Events' 15-year journey had come to a halt, through no fault of my own. On 23rd March, the UK went into lockdown. On the 26th I told the team that with no confirmed projects for the remainder of the year and clients having major doubts for 2021 projects, I couldn't see any way we could continue trading once we'd wrapped up our contractual obligations on cancelled events. I was making them all redundant but requiring them to work their notice, to close down all current projects. It was the worst day of my working life.

The Government had been very honest when it had initiated the lockdown. It had stated that for the following 6-12 months there would be intermittent periods of social distancing. Based on that alone, I couldn't see how clients, sponsors, exhibitors, or attendees would commission and commit to events that could randomly fall into one of those periods and so also have to be cancelled. Likewise, that sort of environment isn't exactly conducive to new business enquiries so I couldn't see the phone ringing off the hook with exciting new, shiny projects.

For me, as hard as it was, the choice I was facing had been very clear. I could have kept the doors open and held out for existing clients to commit to rescheduled events and for new enquiries to come through; whilst hoping the company reserves would outrun the unknown duration of the pandemic. Alternatively, I could wrap up the cancelled events, cease trading and preserve whatever remained of the company reserves. In simple terms, the options were: no company and no funds or no company and some funds. There really wasn't anything in between, so there hadn't been any choice at all.

Furlough (an archaic word that was dusted down as a result of the pandemic) and the business rates grant helped many businesses, but businesses generate far more costs than just 80% of staff salaries. Besides, I needed my staff working to wrap up our projects, so furlough had no relevance to us. The business rates grant barely dented the redundancy costs.

It wasn't lost on me that in some unexpected, bizarre and twisted way, the Universe had shown me a path out of the business; something I'd so desperately needed. Not the way I'd ever wanted or had ever conceived could have happened. I'd wanted to be rewarded for the legacy I'd created and for someone else to build on it. After 15 years, I'd exhausted my vision and energy for the business, so the time had been right to get out, but not at the expense of the team. I was devastated for them. Absolutely beyond gutted. But I had to put myself and my family first. If I'd continued trying to trade, I would have jeopardised their financial stability and future, and after the shit of the previous twelve months, that wasn't something I was prepared to do.

I knew many other businesses had suffered badly and company owners were being crushed by the lack of trading during the early months of the pandemic. To see what was happening all around was truly awful. To many, it was the worst thing that had happened to them, and understandably so. Creating a successful business takes so much more than investing your time and energy. You pour your soul into it. Business coaches tell you it's wrong to think of your business as your *baby*. But how can you not feel like that? It's an extension of yourself. There's a symbiotic relationship: it feeds off you and you feed off it. Helplessly watching it on life support or worse, is agonising.

But my personal perspective was that a global pandemic wiping out the business I'd been investing in for 15 years, over four days, was still only the third worst thing that had happened to me over the previous 12 months. The cardiac arrest and my Mum dying were both 10s on my Shitometer. The business closure could only be a 9. On that basis, I took the view that having already dealt with a couple of 10s, I could somehow handle a 9. Not without consequence, especially to my team, but certainly, in terms of life events, I'd been hit with worse. Much worse. There was also no denying that by ceasing to trade, I'd stumbled across an air pocket. The chance to create that second life I'd felt so robbed of, since November. So, if I was being honest with myself, a 9 was manageable. That said, there was still plenty of work to do.

Whilst large numbers of people (like my team and I) worked through lockdown, the headline story seemed to be the millions of people on furlough being super proactive. The nation's gardens never looked tidier, lofts became more orderly, garages and sheds were dejunked and reimagined to become drinking dens. Then there were the legions who emersed themselves in new activities and challenges: baking banana loaves, learning a musical instrument, teaching themselves Swahili, climbing the equivalent of Everest using only a Viz Annual as a step, completing a marathon by running around a ruler and even, God forbid, doing Joe Wicks keep fit classes in the mornings.

I didn't begrudge these people doing all this fun stuff – they had precious little else to do, but for my team and me, lockdown (or L1, as it was later known) passed us by. We worked all the way through, so yeah, maybe I did begrudge them a bit, as, apart from being at home, winding up the projects was full-on; intense, stressful, and relentless. That was before I even got to managing the company admin and finances. And of course, I had to break the office down. That was another painful process. We'd been in that space 13 years and with 12 workstations, two meeting spaces and storerooms, there was a fair bit of kit to work through. It brought me no joy whatsoever. It took months of sorting, chucking, selling, and giving our world away. So many physical things that had felt so important until so very recently; suddenly, had no value at all. By the end of July, the office had been stripped bare and all trace of it ever being the seat of Team Assured had gone. Then almost immediately, I moved over to Cleethorpes to go through the same process with Mum's house.

There were still aspects of the business requiring my attention daily, so Assured Events remained very much on my mind; even though my efforts bore no fruit and couldn't for the foreseeable future. By the end of August, the final staff; the more senior team on longer notices, had left, leaving only me. My original intention had been to keep the company mothballed so I still had a limited company vehicle with a trading and credit history to develop some hitherto, unidentified business idea. I was hoping the Universe would present opportunities and that by osmosis, the ideas would come to me thick and fast. However, by then, several things had become clear to me. Firstly, even in a mothballed state, the monthly, quarterly, and annual costs associated with keeping a company running, add up. Over 12 months, before even paying myself a low wage, those costs would be a considerable drain on the company reserves.

What's more, despite the hospitality and small events economy opening up, along with the highly popular *Eat Out to Help Out* scheme fuelling heightened public optimism that we'd turned a major corner in the pandemic, there were already governmental and scientific warnings that a second wave was on its way. Historically, second waves in pandemics had usually wrought more damage than the first. The events industry had a *fully open* target date of October 1ˢᵗ, yet it was clear to me, there were very mixed messages in circulation, so I'd never bought into that belief.

But most critically, my appetite to re-engage with the events industry was on the floor. Although, by then, my appetite to engage in anything was questionable. I had no idea what I wanted to do; what I could do, to make a living. I had an overwhelming sense of lethargy and exhaustion and no idea of direction or a drive to find one. I began to wonder about my real motivation for keeping the company going. Was it really that I wanted a limited company vehicle to use for future ventures? Or was it some form of ego, reluctant to let go of a brand I'd built and a name I'd become synonymous with?

Assured Events felt so much a part of my identity. I was the founder and MD of the business and that had been a huge part of my life for a decade and a half. Even if I had no staff and wasn't trading, it was integral to who I was, perhaps even to my status, certainly within the business community; whatever that meant.

If it was ego motivating me to keep Assured Events alive, even if only in name, then I could put a price on that ego – many tens of thousands of pounds a year. Was I prepared to lose that amount of money to placate the attachment I had to the company name I'd built? And for how long? If a second wave was coming, when would it end? The chances were if it did come, we were in for long, dark winter. And if so, how long would it take for business confidence to return? For me, there were too many unknowns, except the price of them.

I concluded that preserving the reserves was worth more than my ego. By late September, the decision had been made to wind up

Assured Events completely. It wasn't taken lightly or as easily as it sounds. It was akin to deciding to take a patient, one that had been close to my heart, off life-support.

## 34

# Back On The Saddle

*"Nothing is permanent in this world. Not even our troubles."*
**Charlie Chaplin**

One of the upsides of the pandemic was that I'd rediscovered road cycling. During the first full lockdown when virtually all shops were closed and millions were working from home, it was wonderful for cyclists as people had nowhere to drive to. The roads were amazingly clear; it must have been what it was like cycling in the 1950s (notwithstanding all the obscenely bright clothing, recording every wheel revolution on Strava and the plethora of gadgets bought from Amazon).

My cycling buddy, for the most part, had been my Brother-in-law, Jus. The first rides in April had left us gasping after 10 miles but by the end of June we were hitting 50 miles, even fitting in a stop for a couple of cans of beer (well, the pubs were still shut!) Our plan for later in the year was to ride coast to coast on *The Way of the Roses* from Morecambe to Bridlington, resurrecting the challenge we'd set ourselves and had intended to complete the previous year - only I'd rather screwed that up. Thanks to the handiwork of my plumber and sparky, Mr D and Gordon along with countless other Doctors, nurses, technicians, follow up checks and medication, I was in great cardiovascular condition and was determined to complete our challenge.

To mark the first anniversary of my cardiac arrest, I'd wanted to do something positive, so decided to cycle into the nearby foothills of the Peak District. One reason was that there are a few sizable speedbumps on a coast to coast, so it was prudent I got some hill training in. But specifically, I wanted to prove to myself, and everyone else, just how far I'd come in the 12 months, since 8<sup>th</sup> May 2019. What I was by then, capable of and how far apart my realities were, between those two dates.

I also wanted to get a picture of me holding my bike aloft, with the city and plains in the background, to email to Gordon and Mr D. I wanted to thank them for all they had done for me and my family, and to show them I was putting their work to good use. The weather had been perfect. It was a lovely ride - very poignant. I'd deliberately wanted to be alone with my thoughts in the hills, reflecting on the previous 12-15 months or so, and felt very grateful for everything everyone had done for me. It wasn't a particularly long ride; only about 20 miles but there had been plenty of huffing and puffing to get up into the hills. The spot on the narrow country lane where I took the timed photo on my phone at bang on 10 am was serenely quiet; just me and the sound of birds and the occasional sheep. I couldn't imagine anything more of a contrast to what had been happening at that very time, one year previously.

There were a few tears, but far more smiles. A big win.

I emailed the image to my Consultants along with a few words and had hoped for, but not expected replies. I felt sure their inboxes would be busy enough without social correspondence from giddy ex-patients cluttering them up, so I was delighted when both responded.

Gordon replied:

*Dear Karl*
*Great to hear from you and I'm delighted to hear that you're doing*
*so well. I've cycled that route a few times so your heart must be doing*
*well to cope with that - did you get to the top of The Pass?*
*With very best wishes to you and your family*

Mr D's secretary replied saying:
*Hi Karl – Mr D sends his very best wishes to you – and says "keep*
*up the good work"*

The replies were wonderful to receive. Reflective of their different characters in some ways but my gratitude will remain undying to them both.

I did reply to each of them with a short note, although no further correspondence was received. But that was irrelevant. I'd closed a big circle.

Jus and I continued to train and were so excited about our road trip. It was set for the week commencing 14<sup>th</sup> September. We'd be getting the train to Morecambe on that Monday; would cycle over the next three days, arriving in Bridlington on the Thursday night and would get the train back on the Friday. We had our accommodation booked and were like two kids looking forward to going on a geography field trip.

With four weeks to go, we hadn't given sponsorship any thought. We were doing this for our own personal enjoyment and the satisfaction of completing the challenge we'd set ourselves a few years prior. I'd also been far too preoccupied with everything else going on with my business and Mum to get involved with organising sponsorship.

But then I did begin to wonder if we should try and raise a few quid for the ward I'd recovered on, to thank them for all their care and support. I'll never be able to fully repay the debt I owe but thought it would show the gratitude I had for them and their work. It just seemed a bit late in the day to start coordinating a social media drive.

That said, I discussed the idea with Jus whilst out on a Sunday ride and we agreed we'd do it. We'd set up a JustGiving page with a target of £500. We had no idea how much we'd raise, but something would be better than nothing.

When we got back to his house, Karina was there, and a BBQ was already sizzling. We shared our decision with our wives and the trip somehow felt even more real. Then Karina said, 'I'm so sorry, I've got some really upsetting news.'

Her face was grave and immediately names started flashing through my mind. I braced myself for impact. Whosever name it was, it was going to be awful.

'Dr A has died.'

I'd been expecting a family name or a friend. It took a second or two to process. I'd always referred to him by his first name.

'Dr A?' The penny dropped. 'Gordon?!'

I was devastated. Confused and devastated. I was choked with emotion. Absolutely gutted.

How could he have died? He was so young – my age! It transpired he'd had a cardiac arrest three weeks prior. It's so unfair that someone who'd spent their entire working life healing heart issues of others should succumb to one himself. Looking back, it feels slightly prophetic, him telling me that he knew my heart better than he knew his own. It appears we'd both been walking time bombs but thanks to Karina's persistence in making a 111 call, I'd been detected and defused.

It immediately cemented our decision to raise funds for the ward and I also dedicated the ride to Gordon on our JustGiving page, thanking him not only for his clinical skills but also for providing the inspiration and belief that I'd be back on my bike again one day.

We completed the ride with all manner of incidents and created memories that will last a lifetime, but they're to be shared another day. We raised over £5000 in three weeks, which blew us away and was incredibly generous of all of those who supported us.

I often still think of Gordon and his words of encouragement. He's also a reminder, as if I ever needed one, that life really is quite short and it can sometimes be a fine line between having one, and not.

# 35

# Smile My Boy. It's Sunrise.

*"Seize the day. Because believe it or not, each and every one of us in this room is one day going to stop breathing."*
**Robin Williams**

The process of closing a solvent company is known as a Members Voluntary Liquidation (let's have a TLA and call it an MVL) and inevitably, was more protracted and required more input than I'd ever realised. It's not just a case of switching off the lights, turning off the website and transferring the funds. Naturally, the closure needed to be advertised in The London Gazette - that well-read business publication - just in case I'd failed to disclose a whole raft of creditors to whom the company owed money to. It all felt rather Dickensian to me. As Charles himself might have said, a fine example of business wiglomeration.

The process also needed to be managed through a liquidations company. This was helpful in the sense that I didn't have the first clue what to do and didn't want to make a costly mistake. Ironically, there are costs attached to avoiding making a costly mistake.

The initial phase took about ten weeks, which I suppose isn't that long but was frustrating when absolutely no money was owed to anyone. In fact, if anything, the company was waiting for a refund from HMRC. By mid-December 2020, 90% of the available funds had been received. The remaining 10% were held back apparently until HMRC had cleared them, along with the refund of Corporation Tax. It's a clichéd certainty as sure as death and taxes that when HMRC wants you to pay said taxes, you get 14 days to sort your shadiz out. When it comes to refunding tax, they apparently need up to a year. I have no idea if that's a Gregorian year, a tax year, a Martian year, or a dog year.

This brings us up to the period when I first began writing in my Begintroduction.

Several other things were contributing to the backdrop of the 2-3 months prior to me starting to write. Namely, the world was once again, going to shit over Covid. Numbers of infections were sky high, and hospitalisations and deaths were on the way up. Eat Out to Help Out was beginning to look like the biggest schoolboy error since the pandemic began and the government had initiated a three-tier local lockdown system.

If you lived in parts of Lancashire, the numbers were rife but if you lived in the Isle of Wight, you were barely aware Covid existed, so it might seem that local variations in lockdowns made sense. Except that it just drove people into lower-tiered areas, So, people living in tier 3 areas where the pubs were shut, would just walk down the road into a neighbouring tier 2 area and get shitfaced in a hostelry overcrowded with their other tier 3 neighbours from the same street. Eventually, tier 4 was introduced and the whole country was pretty much in it apart from Liverpool and Cornwall, which made sense to absolutely no one outside of Liverpool and Cornwall. But at least the lockdowns were managed on a local level.

When I started capturing this stream of consciousness on page one, the country had already begun to slide towards a full lockdown (as we all know, it eventually did) and Christmas was all but cancelled. Except for the 24-26 December, when we were allowed to visit family and The Rona took three days off. Dark days for everyone.

As I write, all of that was almost seven months ago and when I first started to capture my thoughts, I had no plan or idea where it would lead or even for how long I may feel the need to keep writing. There was more than a high chance I'd stop after a few days, just like a new year's resolution fading away, despite all the good intentions. There was no goal or destination; no purpose or reason to keep writing other than a raw need to trawl my mind to try and get to the bottom of my thoughts and feelings at that time.

I'm coming to realise though, the act of downloading these thoughts and feelings, started a process of understanding and to some extent, enlightenment. If you were hoping for a tale of reaching and crossing a finish line, then you're going to be disappointed. I can't even say, 'I'm not there – yet.' I'm not sure if there is a *yet*, or ever will be. It's an ongoing process but I think I'm beginning to get a more authentic understanding, maybe even appreciation of myself and the thoughts and feelings which initiated this whole exercise.

I'll try and explain.

You know how your phone or computer slows down sometimes, and even simple tasks become grindingly painful to complete? That's quite often because there are Apps running in the background, taking up energy and processing capacity. They hog your little machine's ability to work efficiently and effectively. Sometimes you need to upgrade your tech but quite often you just need to manage your Apps better. You don't set them up to work that way. Their activity just creeps up on your phone, slowly draining its ability to do the stuff you want it to do.

That's what was happening to me when I first started typing. I had too many Apps running in the background, and they were messing with my operating system. It sounds counterintuitive given I was wrapping the business up, had no other work to do and therefore had an awful lot of time on my hands. I was entering one of the least busy periods of my entire adult life. Even so, the Apps were whirring in the background.

I can't say specifically what the Apps were, except I now realise they were carrying out some sort of self-assessment and reviewing my connection with the world. We all have these Apps, but at some points in our lives, some of them are busier than others. Mine had been very busy.

When working through the *should I stay or should I go*, of liquidating the business, I mention that I wondered if it had been ego that had been my motivation for keeping it open, albeit mothballed. Once I'd finally decided to liquidate, it had been painful having to change my LinkedIn status; remove my occupation as *Founder and MD*; to post that we were closing for good. I wrote that so much of my identity had been wrapped up in the business and I'd been struggling with letting it go, despite all of the financial arguments being glaringly obvious.

But I've come to realise, it wasn't my ego, as such. It was that I'd become too reliant on Assured Events and my position in it; my ownership of it, as an affirmation of my own self-worth. Let's be clear, we didn't dent the Universe and I'm not saying I was the best MD or decision-maker the world has ever seen – far from it. But none of us is 100% perfect in our private lives, so why should we be in our professional lives? That said, it had been a successful business and that had fed into my self-worth, seemingly far more so, than it should have done.

I'd been struggling with this shredding of affirmation, far more than I'd realised. I'm not proud of it and it sounds, well, *shallow* seems to be the most appropriate word. I could and should have been stronger to take more of my self-worth from my family, friends and other achievements, as a counterbalance to those of my company. It just sort of crept up on me. For as much pain and resentment the business had caused me, there was still a huge pride in having created something from a kitchen table, turning over £2.5M and employing 12, soon to be 16 people. And I had tethered so much of who I thought I was, to that. Or certainly to those achievements.

But as I've worked through this process, I've come to realise, there was an even bigger notion I'd been wrestling with. A different App altogether, but one still grinding away in the background. I couldn't begin to get any clarity on it until about two-thirds of the way through this process and downloading my thoughts through my keyboard. But once the idea had crystalised, I couldn't shake it off and so much of everything that had been rumbling on through my mind began falling into place.

My first life had ended on 8th May 2019. For reasons unknown, I fell into the 8% Club. There had been three days of limbo and successfully coming through the operation on 11th May, marked the beginning of my second life.

A second life? Who would have thought it? Not that I was hoodwinked by the idea I could achieve anything and be anyone I wanted to be. That's just Hollywood bollocks. But I could make changes that would make a big difference to my little corner of the world. I'd had the medium-term hopes of selling the business, and shorter-term plans to reduce my working week, develop personal projects, get back to full strength and live a more rewarding life. I'm paraphrasing, but my second life was going to be more about living a life by design rather than one dictated by a job role. I wanted to do more of what I enjoyed and less of what I didn't. Completely removing the stuff I didn't enjoy would be impossible and was never a goal, but reducing the volume of it seemed achievable.

Within four months of being back at work, that had gone to complete shit. I'd found myself in a worse place than I'd ever been in. I was frustrated that my Shitometer wasn't cutting through. If the worst had already happened to me, why couldn't I shake the feeling of slow, suffocating, resentment?

Then unexpectedly, the Universe had offered me a way out. It was brutal, but an option, nonetheless. It was as if I'd been trapped in a burning building and a *break glass in emergency* button had suddenly appeared in front of me. I realised the only way I could take myself out of the business was to accept the impact of the pandemic, resist attempting to pivot and adapt, and close the doors. There was no guarantee that attempting to adapt would have even succeeded. Failure to succeed would have been costly. Even successfully adapting would have been costly, given the company would still have had to burn through the reserves, for who knew how many months or years.

I hit the button. Although I still had to get out of the burning building, and I had no idea of the route, at least I'd taken the decision to get myself out. By the time I'd started committing these ramblings to keyboard, many months later, I'd pretty much cleared the building, but had absolutely no idea of what was next for me. I still don't. It's quite an unusual position to be in. There haven't been many big career shifts in my life, but when there have been, there was usually a plan. At the time of writing, I have no idea what my *why* is, beyond looking out for my family. I'm not sure what I want to do next or what would fuel my motivation.

We're a big fan of Movie Nights in our house and one of the kids' favourites was the *Night at the Museum* series. There's an exchange of lines towards the end of the third and final film which has always resonated with me, long before I found myself where I do. Probably because it's almost the last line Robin Williams, playing Teddy Roosevelt, ever delivered on film. He shares the scene with Ben Stiller playing Larry, the Museum Security Guard, who's been sacked from the only job he's ever had:

Teddy: You've done your job. It's time for your next adventure.

Larry: [feeling uneasy] I have no idea what I'm gonna do tomorrow.

Teddy: How exciting.

Out of context, it doesn't look much but it always landed with significance, to me. The two characters are looking at the same situation in two completely different ways. Larry had been a Security Guard his whole adult life; it was all he knew. Facing the next day without having to put on that uniform meant addressing the unknown, which was frightening for him. Teddy saw it as an opportunity, a blank canvas and a fresh start, which could only be exciting.

Robin Williams actual final line on film is just a few seconds later: 'Smile my boy. It's sunrise.'

Which now I think about it, is even more poignant. The start of a new day. A new dawn. A new beginning. What isn't there to be excited about?

I've come to realise that in closing the business down, I was effectively closing down my second life. There isn't a date like 8th May, to mark the ending of that life. There will be no anniversary; but the transition of moving on from the working life I'd created, with so much of my self-identity interwoven with Assured Events, means I have a new dawn of my own. I now have the blankest of canvases in front of me - the beginning of my third life.

I realise how self-indulgent and privileged this could sound. But working through this brain dumping process made me realise that, by the time I'd decided to release my Assured team, I was effectively three events behind in processing my own shit. I'd barely scratched the surface of getting my head around my cardiac arrest and subsequent surgery. I'd not properly engaged in the grieving process for Mum and the impact of releasing the team didn't begin to hit me, until the end of 2020. Capturing my thoughts on these pages and addressing these three life events, has helped me considerably.

So, one of the Apps whirring away in the background was the one that had realised my third life had started. Subconsciously I was aware of the new dawn; that I was Larry, facing a new sunrise, but that consciously, I wasn't doing anything about it. This particular App had realised I had no plan, and so my third life was just being frittered away.

Perhaps. But now the notion of starting a third life with *PAUSE* pressed is very much out in the open, I'm more comfortable with it. This is the first time in my life that I've had the opportunity to take a breather. A journey of 30+ working years to where I am today. Some people would love to be in my position – what would they do with it? Retrain? Set up another business? Take a lower-paid, less stressful role somewhere? Volunteer for a charity or community group?

All the above are good uses of time and may yet happen in some capacity. I just don't know in what fields or when, but what I do know is, this period I find myself in, is finite. It's a break between the end of my second life and the start of something new. (I only decided on the title of this tale a few days before completing the first draft, seven months after starting.)

Life is very short; I'm 52 at the time of writing. On average, we only get to orbit the sun 80-ish times. Let's say with a good wind (and I don't stumble on modern life's other tripwires such as Cancer, Parkinson's, Covid, a banal accident or any other potential life shorteners), I somehow make it into my 80s; that's 30-odd summers left. Maybe the last few won't be in the best of health, so what's that - 25 summers? That's not that long. 25 years ago it was Euro '96 and Gazza was making great players look ordinary. That's still pretty fresh in my memory. These next 25 years will pass by just as quickly as the previous 25, so I fully intend to enjoy the years between now and then. To do that, I'll clearly need to be productive. So, there *will* be something else for me; moving on to a new experience. I'm no sloth. I've never been lazy. There will be new opportunities.

That said, I have to say, I've found this writing process very enjoyable. I've not written every day, but when I have, sometimes it's been 500 words and sometimes 5000. It's sometimes been much more challenging than others and all too often I've deleted a load of old guff I'd put down a few days before. But that's OK. I don't regard any of it as a waste of time; even the time spent on the stuff I've deleted. I've enjoyed the process. I've discovered a lot about my own thoughts and feelings: cried a little and laughed a lot, which is probably a good balance for the way to be in life. The 4am demons are partying less often and when they do, they're keeping the noise down to respectable levels and for shorter periods. So, in terms of my whirring background Apps being concerned about me wasting my third life, I'd say I'm far from wasting it. Whilst it's true I'm still not sure of the full plan for my third life, these first few months of it spent writing, have been incredibly rewarding, which is a small and unexpected win. And as a wise young man once told me:

'Any win's a win – and we take them all.'

July 2021

# 36

# The Final Word

*"I may not have gone where I intended to go,*
*but I think I've ended up where I needed to be."*
**Douglas Adams**

It's now October, almost four months since I finished the SFD (Shitty First Draft) of what is the book you're now holding. Having got to the final edit, I felt it just needed a quick update to round the circle before I pressed the *PUBLISH* button.

I remember the joy, elation even, of holding the thick manuscript of around 118,000 words, just about held together by two straining ring clips and thinking, 'Wow. I've done it. I've only gone and written my first book!' Yes, that's right: *First* book. Such optimism!

Once the joy had settled and the box had been emptied of fireworks, I got stuck into my first edit. It was only then I began to realise why they call it the *shitty* first draft. I had no idea how bad some of the writing was. Or how much time it takes or how difficult editing is. And I don't mean copy editing; debating over whether a comma should be here, there or even included at all... although some of that inevitably happened along the way. No. This was about cutting out multiple chunks of copy, huge swathes in some cases. Copy which at some point, I'd felt important enough to write down.

During that first edit, it became apparent that brain dumping thoughts and feelings spanning a short period of my life didn't necessarily translate into a book. So, I had to set about retrofitting these words into something resembling a book. Eventually, I ended up with the (approximately) 97,000 words you've just read. 20,000+ words on the cutting room floor. That's two dissertations. And I remember thinking my (one) dissertation was a massive piece of work.

Then followed the second and third edits. Then the toughest one of all, Karina's feedback. One word: *brutal*. But honest and needed; resulting in more cutting and rewriting of sections followed by a further couple of edits and a copy check. I'd hope if you're still reading by this stage, that you feel I eventually got it somewhere near to *right*. As a debut author, I'd even settle for *just OK*!

To be fair, there's probably a lot more I could've said about some of the events covered, as well as including events that didn't even make the final draft. But in the interests of a quieter, less litigious life, I've consigned those details to the vaults of time.

I also went around the houses about whether to change the names of the people close to me. First, they were in and then I changed them all. But that looked ridiculous and as I thought only people who knew me would buy the book, it'd look ridiculous to them too. So back they changed.

So, what have I been doing in the four months since I finished the SFD and had recognised I was a *Thricer*? Well, aside from the aforementioned editing and rewriting, there was also the crash course in publishing, book marketing and tribe building. All of which would have been impossible without the intervention of Michael Heppell's *Write That Book* programme. (Seriously, if you're even thinking about outing that book that's been bouncing around inside you, look him up.)

In terms of work-work, I'm really enjoying freelancing on various projects, helping smaller businesses become bigger ones. I also have a few exciting ongoing conversations about roles and opportunities which I hope will develop into something more concrete next year.

I'm still in touch with some of my old team and am enjoying watching, and when possible, helping them make a success of going it alone in their own start-up businesses. It's a privilege to be able to help contribute to their journeys. What they've already achieved is phenomenal at a time when the world doesn't know which way is up.

I'm working closely with a local University mentoring some of their second and final year event management students. Apparently *not* owning your own event agency anymore doesn't mean you haven't got experience to share. Good to know and I'm really enjoying it.

Oh, and walking. Lots and lots of hill walking.

So, so far so good. I really hope it continues this way. I've just looked it up and according to the Oxford English Dictionary, *frice* doesn't exist as a word to continue the once, twice, thrice sequence. That scuppers the chance of a sequel if I screw up my *thrice*. Best not do that then.

Crack on!

# 37

# And Just One Or Two Thank Yous…

I have so many people to thank and I don't even know the names of a significant number of them!

I owe an unpayable debt to the Emergency Services Call Handler who talked Karina through CPR the whole time I'd checked out. Without your skills, patience, clarity, and humanity, I wouldn't be here now and my family would be enduring life in the parallel Universe that so plagued me in Chapter 29.

Thank you to the Paramedics who diverted to get to me as quick as was humanly possible and for focussing all their skills and experience so intensely on me. My family and I will always be grateful to you for granting me membership of the 8% Club.

A massive thank you to Mr D and his team for everything you did on 11th May 2019, and the weeks that followed. Your skills and dedication have allowed me to live the active life I so desperately visualised, as I recovered.

To Dr A, Gordon, The Police frontman. It saddens me greatly that you're no longer here. Thank you for giving me the confidence to believe and for inspiring me to *not get in my own way*. I think of your words often.

To Nat and Anita in ICU. You started my post-op journey in the best manner possible. You set the bar high and refused to let me limbo it. And thanks for the drugs. I've never seen grasshoppers that big.

Thank you to all the medical and support staff who supported me across the two hospitals and various wards. Your care and attention were truly appreciated, especially when the journey hit turbulence. Sorry for testing your systems. Keep singing Chiko.

To the young male nurse who provided me with the mission statement: *Any Win's A Win*. You have no idea how profound an impact you had on my life, at the time when I needed it most. That you had no idea you were even doing it tells me you've found your flow in life. Thank you.

To my Assured Events team for doing such a brilliant job during the times I was away from the business. I can imagine the challenges you faced, but not having to worry about *The Shop* gave me the space I needed to recover and I'll always be grateful to you.

To Professor Paul McGee, bestselling author, and performance coach for coming up with the original 1-10 scale. We always enjoyed working with you and implementing your thinking. I hope you can forgive me for adapting and rebranding your scale as my *Shitometer*.

To Michael Heppell, bestselling author, international speaker, and coach for all your advice and guidance provided in the Write That Book Masterclass. You're completely right: '*It's not the book you read that will change your life. It's the one you write.*' This book wouldn't exist if I hadn't joined your programme – thank you.

To everyone on that course who has offered feedback and support, especially my Accountability Group, the phenomenal #ATeam! You're all brilliant and are wonderful authors. You were often the stabilisers on this wobbly bike. I was never on my own

- thank you so much for your advice, guidance, and willingness to share.

Thanks to Nic Crisp, leadership coach and author, for sharing your wisdom and advice early doors on this project. Your encouragement and willingness to share, even after us being out of touch for so long, was greatly appreciated and dispensed at a crucial time.

Thank you to Professor Damian Hughes, international speaker, bestselling author, and co-host of the High Performance Podcast for all of your support. You've inspired me to try and look at challenges differently since the first time we worked together in 2008. But thank you specifically, for initially suggesting I should adapt my ramblings into a book and challenging me when I expressed doubt, when you asked, 'Why not you?' Thanks also for all your ongoing encouragement as this project evolved.

To Jo Shippen, The Queen of Promo, for your unswerving support during testing times and relentless encouragement of this project.

To all my mates who helped me and my family out when I was in hospital and during my recovery; thank you from all of us. We couldn't have done it without you. There are too many to name individually but special mentions go to The Tongues, The Clementis, my Rugby Family, The Abdals, The Cush's, The Turnbulls, the Quizzy Rascals and all their fams.

To my best buddies in Costa del Cleethorpes Darren, Carlos and Taffo, for filling the airwaves with nonsense and keeping the mood light. You're the tonic to my gin.

To Sarah and Jus. Friends first, in-laws second. Thank you for always having our backs but especially so during this journey. We couldn't have gotten through it without you. To lovely Joe for my Iron Man keyring and for always making me laugh.

To Christine for moving in and giving up your own life to help us out in our hours, days, weeks, and months of need. You were a total star. Where would we have been without you? Certainly not in the company of Judge Rinder!

To my big Bro Mark (for being my hero and looking out for me from the beginning of time) & Jayne for both being there with your ever-present support and encouragement, even and especially in the darkest hours. (And who knew Staithes could be Everest's base camp?)

To our sons George and Ben. We're so proud of you. You make us smile every day. You're the reason we kept going; to see you continue to grow into the wonderful, caring, considerate young people you are. We love you with all our hearts.

My greatest thanks of all though, goes to my lovely wife Karina. The cheese to my crackers. The custard to my crumble. The saag to my aloo. Without your composure, focus, strength, energy and determination, we'd all be in Uni#2. Thank you from the bottom of my remodelled heart for the key to the 8% Club and for the gift of every new sunrise in Uni#1. But also, thank you for your bravery in sharing the details of Chapter 13 during the period I was off the grid. I know how difficult it was for you to revisit that time and to share your experiences so publicly in this book. I'm sure your actions will inspire many others to become more cardiac arrest aware and CPR trained. And in doing so, you will have passed on the key to countless other families, so they too will get to enjoy their tomorrows.

Every year over 100,000 people die of Sudden Cardiac Arrest (SCA) in the UK alone. Globally, it claims more lives than colorectal cancer, breast cancer, prostate cancer, influenza, pneumonia, road accidents, HIV, firearms, and house fires combined. This campaign, set up by Arrhythmia Alliance, is working with schools and communities in the UK to build awareness of and provide education and training in CPR as well as the placement of defibrillators.

Every copy of this book sold will generate a donation of £1 to this amazing cause. £1 doesn't sound much compared to the cover price, but ask any self-published author; you're not in it for the money!

So by buying this book, not only will you be rewarded by being highly entertained, but you'll also be entitled to the warm fuzziness of knowing you're contributing to helping communities give others a chance of survival, should an SCA strike.

You can find out more about this lifesaving campaign at www.defibssavelives.org

## About The Author

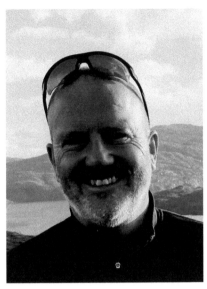

Karl Perry is just a bang average, middle-aged bloke who grew up in Humberston, a small village near Grimsby and Cleethorpes in North East Lincolnshire, but now finds himself living in a similarly small village, south of Manchester.

His educational and early sporting achievements stand out for their lack of being worthy of remark. Something which carried on into early adulthood with his greatest sporting accolade being a second-place go-kart trophy on a stag do.

He currently has absolutely no idea how to describe his occupation, except to say, he seems to have a knack for helping smaller businesses grow a bit bigger. Along the way, he's set up a promotional marketing agency, a property development company, and an event management agency. Only one of these may be still talked about in the present tense.

His playlists rarely leave the 1980s which is reflected in his astonishing dance technique and retention of musical trivia related to the 82-86 era. He doesn't have a dog, which is mentioned for no other reason than he'd really like one, but as compensation, he does feed his neighbour's cat. (In addition to them.)

He's married to Karina, who, when they were students, was attracted to his unique interpretation of céili dancing one St Patricks night, and who has now saved his life, twice. He promises that, should the opportunity ever arise, he's committed to returning the favour.

They have two sons who are legally old enough to have their own families by now but still require feeding, sometimes hourly, so would appreciate it greatly if you purchased this book. Regularly.

**Please get in touch via:**

www.katalystpublishing.com

Twitter: @TheKatalystGuy
Instagram: thekatalystguy